CHARACTERIZATION OF THE T-CELL ACTIVATING

CXC-CHEMOKINE

CXCL11 FROM MAN AND MOUSE

MARTINA MEYER

Die Deutsche Bibliothek – CIP-Einheitsaufnahme
Ein Titeldatensatz für diese Publikation ist bei Der Deutschen Bibliothek erhältlich.

Die Dissertation wurde im Rahmen des FWF Projektes P12872-MED durchgeführt. Wir danken dem Österreichischen Fond "Zur Förderung der Wissenschaftlichen Forschung" für diese Unterstützung.

Herstellung Books on Demand GmbH
ISBN 3-901249-54-0

© 2001 innsbruck university press
Universität Innsbruck, Innrain 52, A-6020 Innsbruck
http://www.university-press.at/

Contents

Abbreviations

A

A_{260}/A_{280}	absorption at 260 / 280 nm
aa	amino acids
ARE	adenylate / uridylate-rich element
aqua d	aqua destillata, distilled water

B

BAC	Bacterial Artificial Chromosome
bp	base pair
BSA	bovine serum albumin

C

CD	cell-surface marker
cDNA	copy DNA / reverse transcribed RNA
Ci	Curie
cpm	counts per minute
CTAB	Hexadecyltrimethyl ammonium bromide
CXC	chemokine of the CXC- subfamily
CXCR3	receptor for CXC-chemokines

D

Da	Dalton
dATP	deoxyadenosine 5´triphosphate
dCTP	deoxycytidine 5´triphosphate
dGTP	deoxyguanosine 5´triphosphate
dTTP	deoxythymidine 5´triphosphate
dNTP	deoxynucleotid 5´triphosphate
ddNTP	di- deoxynucleotid 5´triphosphate
DNA	deoxyribonucleic acid
DNase	deoxyribonuclease
dsDNA	double stranded DNA
DTT	dithiothreitol

E

E.coli	*Escherichia coli*
EDTA	ethylene diamine-tetra acetic acid
ELR	motif of glutamic acid, leucin, arginin
ER	endoplasmic reticulum
EST	expressed sequence tag
EU	endotoxin unit (1.8 EU = 1ng LPS)

F

FCS	fetal bovine serum
FISH	fluorescence *in situ* hybridisation

G

GCG	genetics computer group
GTP	guanosine (-5´-) triphosphate

H

huCXC	human CXC-chemokine
HIV	human immunodeficiency virus type 1

I

IFN-α	interferon-alpha
IFN-_	interferon-beta
IFN-_	interferon-gamma
IL-2	interleukin-2
IPTG	Isopropyl-1-thio-D-galacctoside

K

Kb	kilobase (pair)
kDa	kilodalton

L

LAL	limulus amoebocyte lysate
LB-med	Luria-Bertani medium
LPS	lipopolysaccharides

M

muCXC	murine CXC-chemokine
murine *Scyb*	gene of murine CXC-chemokine
MOPS	morpholinopropane sulfonic acid
Mr	Molecular mass
mRNA	messenger RNA

N

NF-κB	nuclear factor – kappa B
NK cells	natural killer cells
nm	nanometer
NTP	nucleoside triphosphate

O

O.D.	optical density
ORF	open reading frame

P

PAC	P1-derived artificial chromosomes
PCR	Polymerase Chain Reaction
PBMC	peripheral blood mononuclear cells
PBS	phosphate buffered saline
Phe	phenylalanine
PEG	polypropylene glycol
poly-A	polyadenylated mRNA

R

rcf	relative centrifugation force
RNA	ribonucleic acid
RNase	ribonuclease

S

SCYB	CXC-chemokine / gene name
SDS	sodium dodecylsulfate
sDNA	single stranded DNA

T

Taq	Thermus aquaticus
TBE	tris-boric acid + EDTA
7TMR	7 transmembrane receptor
Th1	inflammatory CD4-T-cells
Th2	T helper cells
TNF-_	tumour necrosis factor- alpha
TRIS	Tris-(hydroxymethyl)-aminomethane

U

U	unit
U/µl	unit per µl
UTR	untranslated region
UV-light	ultra violet-light

I. Introduction

1. Definition of chemokines

The function of the immune system depends, to a great extent, on the intercellular communication of effector cells, including T and B-lymphocytes, NK cells, macrophages, dendritic cells and ganulocytes. The successful orchestration of individual responses of effector cell types is mediated by intercellular communication molecules termed cytokines.

The cytokines superfamily is a broad group of signalling proteins including members of the interleukin, interferon, tumour necrosis factor, growth factor, haematopoietic colony-stimulating factors and chemokine family.

Particularly the large families of chemokines and chemokine receptors provide a flexible code for regulating cell traffic and positioning on homeostatic and inflammatory conditions. The complex migratory pathways taken by dendritic cells, T and B cells that are regulated by chemokines and their receptors, provide new insights into the mechanisms that control priming, effector function, and memory responses (Sallusto F et al. 2000).

The name chemokine is a contraction of the words *chemotactic* and *cytokine*. This underlines their connection to the superfamily of cytokines and describes a main function, the chemotaxis.

The chemokine family is defined as low-molecular mass proteins (7-15 kDa), which are structurally related as they share 20 to 70 percent homology in their amino acid sequence.

An important structural feature is the arrangement of the N-terminal cysteine residues, which form disulfide bonds. Chemokines can be divided on account of their cysteine residues into two major and two small subfamilies.

Depending on whether the first two cysteine residues have an amino acid between them or are adjacent, the CXC and the CC family are subdivided. These are the two main families containing nearly all chemokines. The two other subfamilies with only one member found yet for each are the C chemokine(s), lacking cysteine one and three of the typical cysteine structure, and the CX_3C chemokine having three amino acids between the first two cysteine residues (Baggiolini M et al. 1997).

Chemokines fulfil various actions on target cells upon receptor binding. They play important roles in the differential activation, migration and localization of cell types that mediate acute and chronic inflammatory responses. Furthermore, some chemokines were found to function as regulatory molecules in leukocyte maturation and the development of lymphoid tissues. Beyond their effects in the immune system, various chemokines show angiogenic or angiostatic effects. Notably, certain chemokine receptors function as co-receptors for the entry of HIV-1 virus into host cells.

A general description of chemokines and their receptors is given in the first part of the introduction. The second part contains a more detailed description of CXCL11 and a comparison of CXCL11 to the two most related chemokines: CXCL9 and CXCL10.

1.1. Classification and nomenclature

The nomenclature of trivial names still used by many immunologists is sometimes very confusing. The chemokine field is very competitive and often a chemokine was identified at the same time by different groups and was thus assigned different names. CXCL11 (SCYB11) is a perfect example for this difficult nomenclature. It is also termed βR1, H174, SCYB9B, I-TAC or IP-9.

Therefore, a systematic nomenclature was presented at the Keystone Chemokine Symposium 1999, which is based on the structural classification of chemokines in the four subfamilies: CXC, CC, C and CX_3C. These terms are followed by L (for ligand), as all chemokines are soluble factors, mediating their effect via receptor/ligand binding. The ligands of each subfamily are numbered all the way through. The advantage of this new nomenclature is that it directly indicates the class to which each chemokine belongs (Zlotnik A and Yoshie O 2000).

To name the genes of chemokines the Human Gene Nomenclature Committee recommends the SCY nomenclature. SCY is standing for small inducible cytokine and the subfamilies are divided into SCYA, corresponding to the CC subfamily, SCYB, corresponding to the CXC subfamily, SCYC to the C chemokine and SCYD to the CX_3C chemokine. The numbering system is the same as used for the ligands. Thus, genes and gene products still have different systematic names.

In this work, I follow this nomenclature this means that SCYB11 refers to the gene and CXCL11 refers to the mRNA and protein name.

Table 1: List of the known human and mouse chemokines and their systematic nomenclature. This list was adopted from (Zlotnik A and Yoshie O 2000).

Gene name	Ligand name	Initial human term	Initial mouse term
SCYA1	CCL1	I-309	TCA-3 / P500
SCYA2	CCL2	MCP-1 / MCAF	JE
SCYA3	CCL3	MIP-1α / LF78α	MIP-1α
SCYA4	CCL4	MIP-1β	MIP-1β
SCYA5	CCL5	RANTES	RANTES
SCYA6	CCL6	unknown	C10 / MRP-1
SCYA7	CCL7	MCP-3	MARC
SCYA8	CCL8	MCP2	MCP-2
SCYA9/10	CCL9/10	unknown	MPR-2/ CCF18/ MIP-1γ
SCYA11	CCL11	Eotaxin	Eotaxin
SCYA12	CCL12	unknown	MCP-5
SCYA13	CCL13	MCP-4	unknown
SCYA14	CCL14	HCC-1	unknown
SCYA15	CCL15	HCC-2 / Lkn-1 / MIP-1δ	unknown
SCYA16	CCL16	HCC-4 / LEC	LCC-1
SCYA17	CCL17	TARC	TARC
SCYA18	CCL18	DC-CK1/ PARC/ AMAC-1	unknown
SCYA 19	CCL19	MIP-3β/ ELC /Exodus-3	MIP-3β/ ELC/ Exodus-3
SCYA20	CCL20	MIP-3α/ LARC /Exodus-1	MIP-3α/LARC/Exodus-1
SCYA21	CCL21	6Ckine / SLC / Exodus-2	6Ckine /SLC/ Exodus-2
SCYA22	CCL22	MDC / STCP-1	ABCD-1
SCYA23	CCL23	MPIF-1	unknown
SCYA24	CCL24	MPIF-2 / Eotaxin-2	unknown
SCYA25	CCL25	TECK	TECK
SCYA26	CCL26	Eotaxin-3	unknown
SCYA27	CCL27	CTACK / ILC	ALP / CTACK /ILC

Gene name	Ligand name	Initial human term	Initial mouse term
SCYB1	CXCL1	GROα / MGSA-α	GRO / KC
SCYB2	CXCL2	GROβ/ MGSA-β/ MIP-2α	GRO / KC
SCYB3	CXCL3	GROγ/ MGAS-γ /MIP-2β	GRO / KC
SCYB4	CXCL4	PF4	PF4
SCYB5	CXCL5	ENA-78	LIX
SCYB6	CXCL6	GCP-2	CKα-3
SCYB7	CXCL7	NAP-2	unknown
SCYB8	CXCL8	IL-8	unknown
SCYB9	CXCL9	MIG	MIG
SCYB10	CXCL10	IP-10	Crg-2 / IP-10
SCYB11	CXCL11	SCYB9B / I-TAC / IP-9	CXCL11
SCYB12	CXCL12	SDF-1α /β	SDF-1
SCYB13	CXCL13	BLC / BCA-1	BLC / BCA-1
SCYB14	CXCL14	BRAK / Bolekine	BRAK
SCYB15	CXCL15	unknown	Lungkine
SCYC1	XCL1	Lymphotactin / SCM-1α	Lymphotactin
SCYD1	CX3CL1	Fractalkine	Neurotactin

1.2. Chromosome localization

Many chemokines that share structural and functional characteristics are clustered in certain chromosomal locations. Two main clusters have been recognized: one for the CXC chemokines and one for the CC chemokines.

Most of the CC chemokines, which are primarily chemotactic for monocytes, basophils, eosinophils, and lymphocytes are mapped on chromosome 17q11.2. Based on their location in the cluster the CC chemokines can be divided into two groups, the MIP/LD78 group and the MCP group (Nomiyama H et al. 1999).

Most human CXC chemokines, with the exception of CXCL12 (Shirozu et al. 1995), are mapped to the long arm of chromosome 4 (Modi WS and Chen ZQ 1998). Based on their location these CXC chemokines can also be divided into two groups. SCYB1-8 encoding neutrophil chemoattractans are located in a tight cluster on 4q12-4q13, whereas the T-cell chemoattractans SCYB9 - SCYB11 are found in a second mini-cluster separated more than 2 Mb from the main CXC cluster (Tunnacliffe A et al. 1992).

This region on human chromosome 4 is known to be syntenic with mouse chromosome 5. It was shown by Modi WS et al. (1998) that most murine CXC chemokines are assigned to chromosome 5 and further that these genes are also located in two clusters similar to the human ones.

A comparison of CXC-chemokines in man and mouse revealed that huSCYB11, huSCYB10 and huSCYB9 are physically close together on human chromosome 4 and that the murine homologues *Scyb11, Scyb10, Scyb9* are clustered on the orthologous mouse chromosome 5. Beside these striking similarities in the gene localization there are some deviations: Murine *Scyb5* is described to be next to this gene cluster in mouse but is found on a different locus in human. This leads to the suggestion that a translocation of this gene occurred in one of the two species. Another example is SCYB8 that is known from a variety of mammalian species including the guinea pig, but is notably absent in the rat and mouse, indicating an independent gene loss event among muroid rodents.

These findings indicated that although the chemokine gene clusters are well conserved some duplication, loss and translocation events have occurred during mammalian evolution of chemokines (Modi WS et al. 1998). Moreover it is supposed that most if not all chemokines arose from gene duplication of a single ancestral gene (Zlotnik A and Yoshie O 2000).

1.3. Definition of chemokine receptors

Chemokines exert their effects on target cells by signalling through seven transmembrane receptors (7 TMR) coupled to pertussis toxin-sensitive G-protein. This receptor type spans the cell membrane seven times forming four extracellular domains and four intracellular domains. Upon binding their ligand, the receptors initiate intracellular signal cascades that lead to cellular responses. Two of the most widely found intracellular mediators are cyclic AMP and Ca^{2+} (Alberts B 1994).

Generally cellular responses get rapidly attenuated. Mechanisms of signal attenuation include removal of agonist, as well as receptor desensitisation and internalization (Böhm SK et al. 1997). Internalization is described for many CXC and CC chemokine receptors for example for CXCR1 and CXCR2 by CXCL6 ligand binding (Feninger-Barish R et al. 2000). Internalization was also observed for CXCR3 as described in Introduction, chapter 2.7. Down regulation of CXCR3.

1.4. Classification of chemokine receptors:

Chemokine receptors can be divided into several families, including CXC receptors, CC receptors, CX_3C receptors, based on their ligand specificity. But there is also a group of orphan receptors, which are chemokine receptors whose ligands have not been identified yet (Baggiolini M et al.1997).

A special group form chemokine receptors, which are encoded by viruses. For example, human cytomegalovirus encodes a chemokine receptor US28, which binds CCL2, CCL3, CCL4, and CCL5 (Gao JL et al. 1994). ECRF-3, encoded by *Herpesvirus saimiri*, binds CXCL7, CXCL8 and CXCL1 (Ahuja SK et al. 1993).

However, the phylogeny of chemokine receptors, is characterized by two major clusters, one containing CC-chemokine receptors and another containing CXC-receptors as is listed in *Table* 2 (Hughes AL and Yeager M 1999).

Table 2: List of human chemokine receptors and their ligands. This list was adopted from (Baggiolini M. 1998).

Receptors	Ligands
CXCR1	IL-8, GCP-2
CXCR2	IL-8 and all ELR-containing CXC chemokines
CXCR3	CXCL9, CXCL10, CXCL11
CXCR4	SDF-1
CXCR5	BCA-1, BCL-1
CCR1	MIP-1α, RANTES, MCP-3
CCR2 a/b	MCP1-4
CCR3	Eotaxin, RANTES; MCP2-4
CCR4	TARC, MDC
CCR5	MIP-3, RANTES, MIP-1β
CCR6	MIP-3α
CCR7	MIP-3β, SLC
CCR8	I-309
XCR1	Lymphotacin
CX$_3$CR1	Fractalkine

A remarkable feature of the chemokine receptor superfamily is their promiscuity for ligand binding. As is shown in *Table 2*, most chemokine receptors recognize more than one chemokine and several chemokines bind to more than one receptor. In general the chemokine subfamily integrity is maintained, as the promiscuous binding to receptors occurs within one subfamily (Gale JL and McColl SR 1999).

However, latest findings suggest that the natural ligands for CXCR3 could act as an antagonist for CCR3 (Loetscher P et al. in press), which is described in more details in Introduction, <u>chapter 2.6.4. CCR3 down-regulation by CXCL11, CXCL9 and CXCL10</u>.

1.5. General effects of chemokines acting via their receptors

Depending on function and pathophysiological roles, it is possible to distinguish between inflammatory and homing chemokines. Inflammatory chemokines are produced under pathological conditions by tissue cells and infiltrating leukocytes. The production is strongly induced by cytokines and bacterial toxins.

However, constitutively expressed chemokines seem to fulfil housekeeping functions. They may be involved in leukocyte maturation in the bone marrow, the traffic and homing of lymphocytes and the mechanisms of leukocyte circulation.

1.5.1. Receptor-ligand binding

Receptor recognition depends on structural motifs located at the N-terminal region of the chemokines. Extensive structure-activity studies have led to the proposal of a two-step interaction of the chemokines with its receptors (Loetscher P et al. 1998). It is supposed that the initial step involves an interaction with a site in the loop region of the ligand that follows the CXC or CC motif. This exposes the receptor site and allows the subsequent binding of the N-terminal region to a buried site in the receptor (Clark-Lewis I et al. 1994, Crump MP et al. 1997).

The receptor activating effect was especially shown for the ELR motif. It was demonstrated by selective deletion that the amino acid sequence Glu-Leu-Arg (ELR motif) contributes to high-affinity binding and that this motif is the receptor triggering part of the molecule. The ELR motif is conserved at the NH_2 end of all CXC-chemokines which bind on CXCR1 and CXCR2 and act on neutrophils (Clark-Lewis et al. 1991).

However, the ELR motif alone is not sufficient for receptor binding, as linear and cycling ELR-containing oligopeptides neither bind to the receptors nor stimulate them (Clark-Lewis I et al. 1993). It is believed that a core domain of the protein determines receptor binding selectively and facilitates the access of the ELR motif to the receptor triggering site (Baggiolini M et al. 1997).

Another characteristic of the ELR motif is its angiogenic effect, which is described in Introduction, <u>chapter 1.5.4. Angiogenic and angiostatic effects of CXC chemokines.</u>

The importance of the ELR motif has led to a subdivision of CXC chemokines into ELR containing and non-ELR containing chemokines.

1.5.2. Chemotaxis

In chemotaxis, cells move in the direction of increasing concentration of a chemoattractant, which is typically a soluble molecule that can diffuse from the site of its production where its concentration is highest (Devreotes PN and Zigmond SH 1988). Leukocytes, which can sense a concentration difference of 1 % across their diameter, move steadily in the direction of the chemoattractant (Springer TA 1994).

Beside the effect of leukocyte recruitment to sites of inflammation, chemokines are capable to increase adhesion of leukocytes to endothelial cells and to stimulate transendothelial migration. The adhesion and migration through blood vessels includes several (reversible) steps (Butcher EC and Picker LJ 1996). Primary adhesion, which is transient and reversible in seconds, brings the leukocyte in contact with the vessel wall. In the second phase the leukocyte gets activated by various factors (e.g. chemokines) before an activation dependent „arrest" between leukocyte and endothelial cell occurs. In the final step the cell migrates between endothelial cell junctions into the extracellular matrix of the tissue.

Leukocytes generally express several types of chemokine receptors. These are required to perform distinct steps in the process of extravasation and positioning within the tissue (Salusto F et al. 2000). For instance a multistep navigation was shown for neutrophils which can migrate effectively to a secondary distant agonist after migrating up the primary gradient into a saturation, non-orienting concentration of an initial attractant (Foxman EF et al. 1997).

1.5.3. Intracellular calcium release

The binding of extracellular signalling molecules to cell-surface receptors causes the release of Ca^{2+} from the endoplasmic reticulum (ER). The concentration of free Ca^{2+} in the cytosol of cells is very low ($<10^{-7}$ M), whereas its concentration in the extracellular fluid and in the ER is high ($\sim 10^{-3}$ M). When a signal transiently opens Ca^{2+} channels in either of these membranes, Ca^{2+} is released into the cytosol, where it triggers Ca^{2+}-responsive proteins (Alberts B et al. 1994). The increase of intracellular Ca^{2+} is one of the earliest events occurring in response to the binding of chemokines to their receptors.

1.5.4. Angiogenic and angiostatic effects of CXC chemokines

The presence or absence of the ELR motif in CXC chemokines functionally defines the angiogenic or angiostatic characteristics of chemokines (Baggiolini B et al. 1989). Angiogenesis is characterized as the new formation of blood vessels, an event involved in numerous physiological processes, such as embryonic development, chronic inflammation and the growth of malignant solid tumours.

It was demonstrated that CXC chemokines that contain the ELR motif, but not those that lack these three amino acids (CXCL4, CXCL9 and CXCL10 and the later found CXCL11), are potent inducers of angiogenic activities. Moreover, an insertion of ELR into CXCL9 generated a protein with angiogenic effects, while the mutation of the ELR motif in IL-8 turned the protein into an angiostatic factor (Strieter RM et al. 1995).

1.6. Role of chemokine receptors in HIV-1 infection

The entry of HIV-1 into host cells is a multistep process. The HIV-1 virus is surrounded by a lipid membrane, which protrudes the virally encoded env glycoprotein. The env-protein mediates the binding of virus to the cell surface through binding to $CD4^{+}$, the primary virus receptor (Horuk R. 1999).

However, the subsequent interaction with a chemokine receptor, which functions as a co-receptor, is necessary for fusion between the viral and the cellular membrane. CCR5 and CXCR4 belong to the chemokine receptors helping the virus to enter the cell.

CXCR4 is described to act as a co-receptor required for entry by T lymphocyte tropic (T tropic) virus strains, while CCR5 is an entry cofactor for monocyte / macrophage tropic (M tropic) HIV-1 strains (Mellado M et al. 1998).

CCL2, CCL3, CCL4 and CCL5 (the natural ligands for CCR5) are detected to be potent inhibitors of infection by M-tropic HIV strains, while CXCL12 was found to be a potent inhibitor of infection by T tropic HIV-1 strains (Gong W et al. 1997, Bleul CC et al. 1996).

The discovery that chemokine receptors are co-receptors for HIV-1 infection opens the door for novel antiviral approaches, using specific chemokine receptor antagonists, which could block the binding and subsequent entrance of HIV-1 virus into the cell membrane (Horuk R. 1999).

2. Common characteristics of the related chemokines CXCL9, CXCL10 and CXCL11 in man and mouse

2.1. Identification of CXCL10 and CXCL9

The murine and human cDNAs of CXCL10 and CXCL9 were all identified as IFN-γ inducible transcripts:

CXCL10 (also named IP-10 for IFN-γ inducible protein, 10 kDa) was discovered first by differential screening of a cDNA library prepared from a lymphoma cell line (U937) treated with recombinant IFN-γ (Luster AD et al. 1985). The cDNA encodes for a precursor protein of 98 amino acids (Mr 10.855) with a 21 amino acid signal peptide, leading to secretion of a 77 amino acid mature protein (Mr 8.620) (Sarris AH et al. 1995).

CXCL9 (also named MIG for monokine induced by IFN-γ) was isolated by screening a cDNA library from lymphokine-activated macrophages and identified as an mRNA selectively induced in response to IFN-γ. The cDNA encodes for a 125 amino acid protein (Mr 14.019) containing the 22 amino acid signal peptide. Therefore the secreted mature protein is predicted for 103 amino acids (Mr 11.725) (Farber JM. 1990).

MuCXCL9 (also named muMIG) (Farber JM 1990) and muCXCL10 (also termed CRG-2 derived from cytokine–responsive gene) (Vanguri P and Farber JM 1990) were both discovered in a collection of 11 genes identified by differential screening of a cDNA library prepared from a mouse macrophage cell line (RAW264.7) that had been treated in the presence of cycloheximide, with supernatants from concanavalin A-stimulated splenocytes (Farber JM. 1992). The mouse CXCL10 cDNA encodes a protein of 98 amino acids (Mr 10.781), and the secreted protein is predicted to have 77 amino acids (Mr 8.700) (Vanguri P and Farber JM 1990). For murine

CXCL9 cDNA the respective length is126 amino acids (Mr 14.461) and 105 amino acids (Mr 12.193) (Farber JM 1992).

2.2. Identification of CXCL11

Human CXCL11 was cloned by several groups and reported under different names. Because this can lead to some confusion, partial and full-length cDNA sequences isolated from various cellular sources are summarized here.

The first partial cDNA was isolated by RNA fingerprint from an IFN-γ-stimulated astrocytoma cell line and was named β-R1 (Rani MSR et al. 1996). This newly found mRNA was strongly upregulated upon induction with IFN-γ and IFN-β. A year later, a partial cDNA sequence was isolated from activated PBMC by a new technique selecting cDNAs which encode a signal peptide. The cDNA named H174 was described to be a homologue to huCXCL9 (Jacobs KA et al. 1997).

In 1998, the complete cDNA of this CXC-chemokine named I-TAC (interferon-inducible T cell alpha chemoattractant), isolated from cytokine-activated human astrocytes was published (Cole KE et al. 1998). The mRNA expression in different tissues was investigated showing a high expression in peripheral blood leukocytes, pancreas, and liver, followed by thymus, spleen, and lung. Furthermore, it was demonstrated that the chemically synthesized CXCL11 peptide binds selectively to the CXCR3 receptor and initiates intracellular calcium influx and chemotaxis.

In the same year the chromosomal localization of this chemokine (named SCYB9B) at chromosome 4q21.2 was described by our group (Erdel M et al. 1998). In the following year we published the structure of the SCYB11 gene and characterized a cDNA clone from IFN-γ-treated human myelomonocytic cells (THP-1). In addition, we determined the mRNA expression of CXCL11 upon IFNs in THP-1 cells and the expression pattern in various human cell lines (Laich A et al. 1999).

At the same time the native protein was isolated from supernatant of IFN-γ-stimulated keratinocytes by binding to the CXCR3 receptor expressed on transfected

CHO-K1 cells (Tensen CP et al. 1999a). In a second paper published the same year, the genomic organization and a computer assisted analysis of the promoter region were published (Tensen CP et al. 1999b).

Recently, we isolated the homologous murine cDNA from IFN-γ / LPS-stimulated RAW264.7 mouse macrophage-like cells and clarify genomic organization and chromosomal localization (Meyer M et al. 2000). The murine cDNA was also identified in search for glucocorticoid-attenuated response genes. This group investigated also the murine CXCL11 expression pattern in multiple tissues during endotoxemia (Widney DP et al. 2000).

2.3. Peptide data of CXCL11

The reading frame of human CXCL11 encodes for a 94 amino acid protein containing a putative 21 amino acid signal peptide, characteristic for secretory proteins. The mature protein is likely to consist of 73 amino acids (Laich A et al. 1999). The molecular mass of the mature protein was found to be 8303 Da, as was determined for the native protein, isolated from the supernatant of keratinocytes stimulated with IFN-γ (Tensen CP et al. 1999a).

The reading frame from murine CXCL11 encodes a 100 amino acid precursor protein containing also a putative signal peptide of 21 amino acids. Thus the mature protein is likely to consist of 79 amino acids (Meyer M et al. 2000). The molecular mass of the mature protein after folding via two disulphide bonds is 9109. The theoretical mass was confirmed for the recombinantly expressed muCXCL11 chemokine by electrospray ionization mass spectrometry (Hensbergen PJ et al. in prep.).

2.4. Expression of CXCL11, CXCL9 and CXCL10 mRNA

Human

IFN-γ was the most potent inducer of CXCL11 mRNA as compared with IFN-α and IFN-β in THP-1 cells as was detected by Northern blot experiments (shown in *Figure 1*). The effect of all three IFNs was enhanced by combination with LPS or TNF-α. As a single stimulus, TNF-α and LPS had no effect on the induction of CXCL11 mRNA.

Various human cell types and cell lines were identified to express CXCL11 mRNA upon treatment with IFN-γ, including HUVEC and fibroblasts (Laich A et al. 1999), although the expression pattern in THP-1 cells could not be generalized to other cell types. For example in dermal fibroblasts the signal was detectable only when IFN-γ and LPS were combined, whereas a single stimulus did not induce detectable amounts of CXCL11 mRNA (Laich A et al. 1999). Furthermore, IFN-β alone was a strong inducer in human astrocytoma cells, whereas IFN-α was only a weak stimulus (Rani MRS et al. 1996).

Studies on CXCL9 and CXCL10 showed similar expression patterns. The most potent inducer of CXCL10 in macrophage cell lines and monocytes is IFN-γ, although other agents like IFN-α, IFN-β and LPS are also effective (Luster AD et al. 1985). As a single stimulus, IFN-γ induced CXCL11 in macrophages, keratinocytes and fibroblasts (Tensen CP et al. 1999b, Laich A et al. 1999), whereas the combination of IFN-γ and TNF-α induced expression of CXCL9 in endothelial cells (Ebnet K et al. 1996).

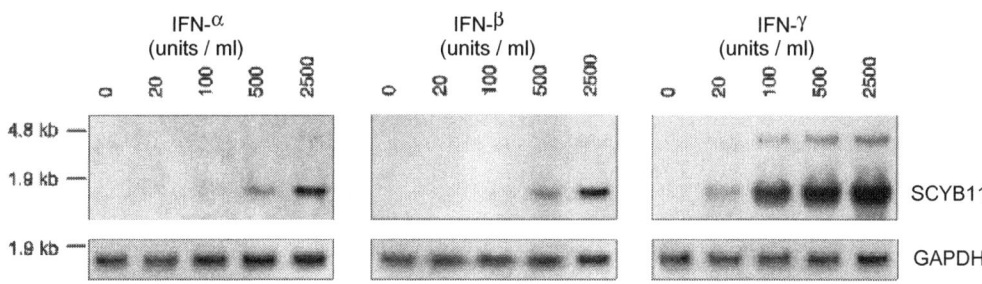

Figure 1: Expression pattern of CXCL11 mRNA in THP-1 cells

THP-1 cells were treated with various doses of IFN-α, IFN-β and IFN-γ for six hours. The Northern blot was hybridized with the entire coding region of CXCL11. The *Figure* is adopted from (Laich A et al. 1999).

Murine

Similarly to the expression of human CXCL11 in human cells, murine CXCL11 is induced in murine macrophage like cell lines, in fibroblasts and in dendritic cells by various stimuli. The relative potential of interferons to induce murine CXCL11 in RAW264.7 cells was IFN-γ > IFN-β > IFN-α, but IFN-β alone was also a strong stimulus. A very similar expression pattern was also observed for induction of muCXCL9 and muCXCL10. *Figure 2A* shows the induction of muCXCL9, muCXCL10 and muCXCL11 in the macrophage like cell line RAW264.7 upon stimulation with IFN-α, IFN-β, and IFN-γ. The half maximal effective concentration (EC_{50}) of interferons for the induction of murine CXCL9, CXCL10 and CXCL11 mRNA expression is shown in *Figure 2B*. IL-1β and TNF-α had only weak effects on expression of all three chemokines, while LPS was generally a moderate inducer.

Constitutive muCXCL9, muCXCL10 and muCXCL11 mRNA expression was observed in several cell types tested. IFN-γ given as a single stimulus increased all three chemokine mRNA levels up to 10000-fold. The expression levels of muCXCL11, muCXCL9 and muCXCL10 were comparable in cell lines upon induction with IFN-γ.

The mRNA expression patterns in mouse were quantified by real-time PCR (Meyer M et al. submitted).

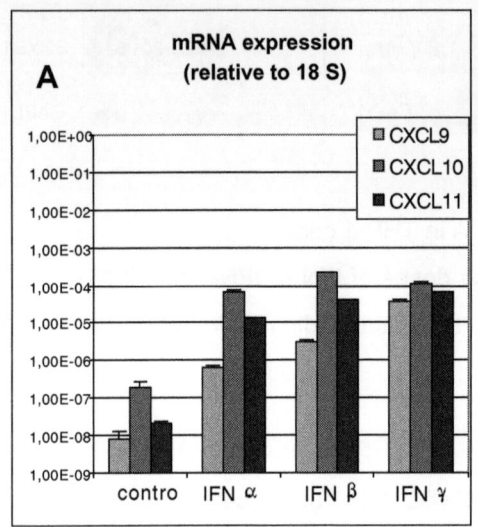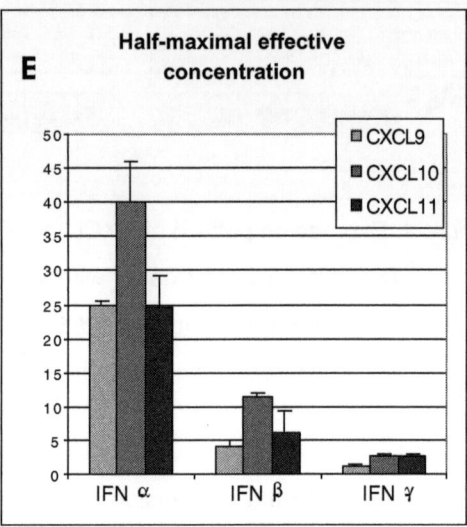

Figure 2: Comparison of the mRNA expression of CXCL9, CXCL10 and CXCL11 in response to various interferons.

A: RAW264.7 cells were treated for 6 hours with 500 U/ml of IFN-α, IFN-β, or IFN-γ.

B: Half-maximal effective concentration of interferons for induction of CXCL9, CXCL10 and CXCL11 mRNA expression. RAW264.7 cells were treated with various doses (from 2 to 500 U/ml) of interferons for 6 hours and the EC_{50} was estimated by plotting IFN-dose versus mRNA level. Values were taken from Meyer M. et al. submitted.

2.5. Expression of CXCR3

CXCR3 is a 7-transmembrane G-protein coupled receptor (7 TMR) highly specific for CXCL10, CXCL9 (Loetscher P et al. 1997) and the later identified CXCL11(Cole KE et al. 1998, Tensen CP et al. 1999a). Northern blot analysis indicated that CXCR3 is mainly expressed on activated T cells (Loetscher P 1996). Moreover a small proportion of circulating blood T-cells, B cells and natural killer cells also express CXCR3 (Qin S et al. 1998). CCR5 shows a similar expression pattern as CXCR3. These two chemokine receptors appear to be markers for T cells associated with certain inflammatory reactions.

Moreover it was shown that CXCR3 and CCR5 are preferentially expressed in human Th1 cells. In contrast Th2 cells preferentially express CCR4 and CCR5. It was suggested that the differential expression of chemokine receptors might orchestrate the migration and tissue homing of Th1s and Th2s (Bonecchi R et al. 1998).

The murine homologue of human CXCR3 receptor was cloned from a Th1-lymphocyte library, shown to be 86 % identical to the human receptor. The murine homologue shows a similar expression pattern as its human counterpart (Lu B et al. 1999).

2.6. Biological activities of CXCL11, CXCL10 and CXCL9

To characterize the biological activity of chemokines and their receptors the chemotaxis assay and the calcium mobilization assay are widely used.

The chemotactic activity can be measured by selective movement of cells through a filter (3 to 10 µm pore size) towards the chemoattractant. To detect the change of intracellular Ca^{2+} levels, target cells are loaded with a calcium-binding fluorescence dye i.e. Fura-AM. After loading, cells are incubated with a chemokine. The change of fluorescence intensity can be measured.

2.6.1. Chemotaxis

Human

Chemotaxis assays performed with cells transfected with human CXCR3 receptor and with IL-2 activated T memory cells (Cole KE et al. 1998, Laich A et al. 1999, Tensen CP et al. 1999a) demonstrated that human CXCL11 induces a potent chemotactic response. The chemotaxis peaked at 10 nM and decreased at higher concentrations, in a typical bell-shaped chemotactic response curve.

As described in Introduction, chapter 1.5.1. Receptor-ligand binding, the N-terminus of the chemokines is most important for receptor binding and activation. This was also shown for CXCL11. The chemotactic potency of recombinant human CXCL11 gets lost if the N-terminus is truncated by removing the first two amino acids (Hensbergen PJ et al. in prep).

Comparison of the chemotactic potency of CXCL11 showed that CXCL11 is a better chemoattractant than CXCL9 and CXCL10. Twice as many cells migrated in response to 10 nM CXCL11 than to 10 nM CXCL10 (Cole KE et al. 1998, Tensen CP et al. 1999a). Therefore it was concluded that CXCL11 is the dominant ligand for this receptor (Tensen CP et al. 1999a).

Murine

Chemotactic activity of muCXCL11 was confirmed using murine pre B 300-19 cells transfected with muCXCR3. Murine CXCL11 was shown to be a more potent chemotactic protein showing an optimum at 3 nM, as compared to 30 nM for muCXCL10 and 100 nM for muCXCL9. Murine CXCL11 was also a chemoattractant for human T cells, although its threshold concentration was about 30 times higher relative to human CXCL11 (Meyer M et al. submitted).

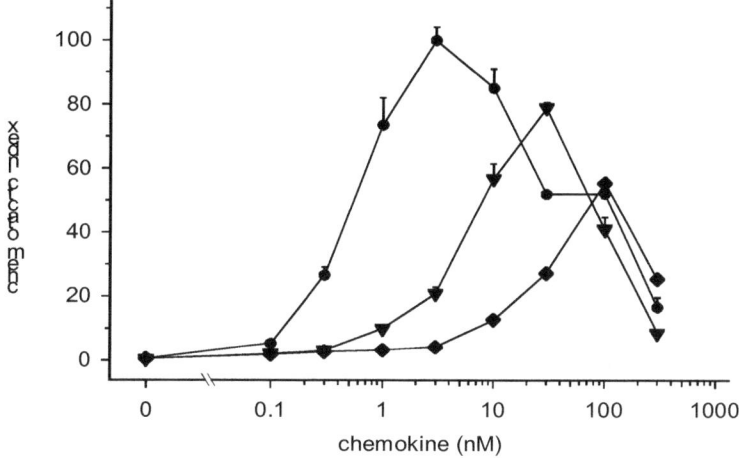

Figure 3: Chemotactic activity of murine CXCL11 in comparison to muCXCL9 and muCXCL10.

Migrated 300-19 pre-B cells, transfected with murine CXCR3, in response to muCXCL9 ♦, muCXCL10 ⌐, and muCXCL11 ●, were quantified by fluorescence detection. Chemotaxis is expressed as chemotactic index in relation to cell counts obtained by 3 nM murine CXCL11, respectively, set to 100. Graphic was adapted from Meyer et al. (submitted.)

2.6.2. Calcium mobilization

Human

Human CXCL11 induced a rapid and transient increase in intracellular Ca^{2+} levels in a dose-dependent manner with peak activity at 10 nM. CXCL11 is ~100 fold more potent in activation of CXCR3 expressed on transfected CHO cells as compared with recombinant CXCL10, and 1000-fold more active than recombinant huCXCL9 (Tensen CP et al. 1999a).

Furthermore, CXCL11 is much more active in cross-desensitation of chemokine-induced Ca^{2+} mobilization in transfected CHO cells. 1 nM CXCL11 inhibited CXCL10 (10 nM) or CXCL9 (100 nM) responses, whereas 1 nM CXCL11 generated a response after previous activation by 10 nM CXCL10 or 100 nM CXCL9 (Tensen CP et al. 1999a).

Murine

Ca^{2+} mobilization experiments using CHO cells transfected with CXCR3 showed a maximum response at 30 nM CXCL11.

300 nM of muCXCL9 and of CXCL10 resulted in a Ca^{2+} signal comparable to that obtained by 10 nM of CXCL11. Furthermore CXCL11 evoked not only a Ca^{2+} signal via the murine CXCR3 receptor but also via the human CXCR3 receptor. Cross desensitization studies demonstrated that muCXCL11 stimulated muCXCR3 at much lower doses than muCXCL9 or muCXCL10. Furthermore, muCXCL11 completely inhibited the Ca^{2+} mobilization induced by muCXCL9 and muCXCL10, while muCXCL9 and muCXCL10 did not completely block the signals evoked by murine CXCL11 (Meyer M et al. submitted).

2.6.3. Adhesion mediated by CXCL10, CXCL9 and CXCL11

CXCL10 and CXCL9 were shown to induce rapid and transient adhesion of IL-2 stimulated T lymphocytes to immobilized integrin ligands through their receptor CXCR3. This integrin-mediated adhesion to the vascular endothelium is an essential step in leukocyte diapedesis. Both chemokines, CXCL9 and CXCL10 are produced in human umbilical vein endothelial cells (HUVEC) (Laich A et al. 1999) upon stimulation with IFN-γ and TNF-α. In contrast, an anti-CXCR3 monoclonal antibody treatment caused arrest and firm adhesion (Piali L et al. 1998).

Furthermore, it was shown that the chemokines CXCL11, CXCL9 and CXCL10 could also play a critical role in the recruitment and retention of activated T cells in atherosclerosis. This was suggested as an analysis of human atherosclerotic plaques showed a coexpression of the chemokines CXCL10, CXCL9, CXCL11 and their common receptor CXCR3 in the lesions (Mach F et al. 1999).

2.6.4. CCR3 down-regulation by CXCL11, CXCL9 and CXCL10

The ligands of CXCR3 receptor CXCL11, CXCL9 and CXCL10 are natural antagonists for CCR3. This be came clear recently as these three chemokines competed for the binding of eotaxin to CCR3 and inhibited migration and Ca^{2+} influx. They could inhibit migration and Ca^{2+} changes induced in CCR3 expressing cells. Furthermore, none of the antagonistc induced internalization of CCR3 indicating that they lack agonistic effects and thus qualify as pure antagonists (Loetscher P et al. in press).

This finding suggests that chemokines that attract Th1 cells via CXCR3 can concomitantly block the migration of Th2 cells in response to CCR3 ligands, thus enhancing the polarization of T-cell recruitment. The selective responsiveness of T-cell subsets to chemokines is described in Introduction, chapter 2.5. Expression of CXCR3 receptor.

2.7. Down-regulation of CXCR3

Memory / effector T cells could transiently switch chemokine receptor expression upon T-cell stimulation. First after binding of inflammatory chemokines (like CCR5 and CXCR3) the receptor gets rapidly down-regulated. This occurs within 6 hours after ligand binding. Subsequently, receptors for constitutive chemokines are transiently up-regulated for 2 to 3 days. This loss of responsiveness to inflammatory chemokines induced by antigenic stimulation may result in a migratory arrest for activated T cells and may allow these cells to sense new chemotactic gradients (Sallusto F et al. 1999).

CXCR3 down-regulation was also shown to occur during continuous, long-term exposure of cells to receptor agonists. A high dose of CXCL11 induced a fast and strong internalization of CXCR3 on activated CD4[+] T cells and CXCR3 transfected 300-19 cells. CXCL10 and CXCL9 induced a less strong decrease of CXCR3 (Sauty A et al. 1999).

2.8. Anti-tumour effect of CXCL9 and CXCL10

Chemokines, lacking the ELR motif (e.g. CXCL4, CXCL10 and CXCL9), are angiostatic and can induce tumour regression by reducing the blood supply. This was shown in mice for CXCL10, CCL5 and CCL1.

Sgadari C et al. (1997), showed that inoculation of purified recombinant human CXCL9 or CXCL10 consistently caused tumour necrosis associated with extensive vascular damage. Also the anti-tumour effect of IL-12 is associated with the chemokines CXCL9 and CXCL10. The local and systemic treatment with IL-12 caused an upregulation of IFN-γ, CXCL10 and CXCL9 gene expression in the tumour. Levels of CXCL10 and CXCL9 expression in the tumour, the liver and the kidney correlated inversely with tumour size. Thus, CXCL10 and CXCL9 contributed to the antitumoural effect of IL-12 through their inhibitory effects on tumour vascularisation (Kanegane C et al. 1998).

II. Methods

1. Application of bacterial cells

E.coli and its strains like XL-1 (used for this work) are wide-spread tools in molecular biology to generate large amounts of target DNA sequences. *E.coli* is a rod-shaped bacterium (Gram-negative) with a circular chromosome that could carry extrachromosomal DNA molecules called plasmids.

Bacterial plasmids are frequently used in cloning protocols to generate DNA fragments of interest. They are self-replicating, circular and can easily be isolated from the *E.coli* host cell. Plasmid DNA is introduced into the host cell by transformation, like the calcium chloride method used in this work.

1.1. Culturing of bacterial cells

E.coli strains were generally grown on complete medium. As a solid medium LB-agar plates were used. Liquid cultures were grown in LB or TB-medium. If the cells were transformed with a plasmid vector, an antibiotic was supplied to the LB-agar, because all plasmid vectors used in this work carry an antibiotic resistance (listed in *Table 3*).

Table 3: Plasmid vectors used in this work and their antibiotic resistance.

Plasmid vector	Antibiotic	Concentration
pBluescript SK$^-$	ampicillin	50 µg/ml
TOPO^{TM}TA Cloning	kanamycin	50 µg/ml
PAC	kanamycin	25 µg/ml
BAC	chloramphenicol	12,5 µg/ml
pGL3$_{basis}$	ampicillin	50 µg/ml
pGL3$_{promoter}$	ampicillin	50 µg/ml
pRL-TK	ampicillin	50 µg/ml
pET-32a	ampicillin	50 µg/ml

1.2. Preparation of competent cells

Cells used for transfection were made competent with calcium chloride. XL-1 cells were spread out on LB-agar plates and incubated at 37 °C over night. A single colony was inoculated in 25 ml LB-medium and incubated at 37 °C in a shaker over night. On the next day, 5 ml from the pre-culture was transferred to 500 ml LB-medium in an Erlenmeyer flask and shaken at 37 °C until the A_{620} reached 0.45-0.55. Cells were chilled immediately in ice water for 2 hours and subsequently collected by centrifugation at 2000 rcf for 20 min at 4 °C. Cells were resuspended in 15ml ice-cold trituration buffer and then diluted to 500 ml with the same solution.

To make a glycerol stock culture of competent cells, cells were further incubated for 45 min on ice and then centrifuged at 2000 rcf for 10 min and gently resuspended in 50 ml ice-cold trituration buffer. Glycerol was added drop wise until a final concentration of 15 % (V/V) was reached.

1.3. Transformation with calcium chloride

100 µl competent cells were gently mixed with 50 µl 100 mM calcium chloride in a 1 ml tube and placed on ice before 1 µl purified plasmid DNA was added. The competent cells were stored for one hour on ice before they were shock-heated by placing the tube for 2 min in a 42 °C water bath. Subsequently, cells were placed back on ice and 1 ml LB-broth was added. The transfected cells were incubated for 2 hours at 37 °C on a shaker before they were spreaded out on an appropriate antibiotic-containing LB-agar plate. Plates were incubated over night in at 37 °C.

2. Isolation of plasmid DNA

2.1. Mini preparation (CTAB)

Over night culture

20 ml TB-medium was transferred to a 50 ml, sterile tube and antibiotic was supplied in the required concentration. A single bacterial colony was picked from the plate with an inoculation needle. The tube was incubated at 37 °C in a shaker over night. Cells were harvested by centrifugation at 3300 rcf for 30 min at 4 °C.

Preparation

The over night culture was centrifuged for 30 min at 3300 rcf. The cell pellet was resuspended in 1.3 ml ice cold STET solution by pipetting several times up and down. 40 µl lysozyme solution was added and incubated for 10 min at room temperature. This cell lysate was boiled for 3 min in a water bath, then immediately placed on ice and subsequently centrifuged by 13000 rcf at 4 °C for 30 min.

The supernatant was transferred into a new 1.5 ml tube. To destroy RNA, 10 µl RNase A solution (10 µg/µl) was added and incubated for 15 min at 37 °C.

CTAB-binding

Subsequently, 100 µl CTAB solution were added and incubated for 20 min at room temperature. After incubation, the DNA bound to CTAB was centrifuged at 25 °C and 13000 rcf for 5 min at room temperature. Subsequently, another 100 µl CTAB solution was added, incubated for 20 min again, and centrifuged for 5 min at 13000 rcf at 25 °C. The supernatant was removed and the pellet resuspended in 400 µl ice-cold 1.2 M NaCl solution. After a further step of centrifugation (5 min at 13000 rcf and 4 °C), the supernatant was transferred to a new 1.5 ml tube. For precipitation, 1 ml ethanol was added, the sample was vortexed and incubated at -20 °C over night. DNA was collected by centrifugation and washed with 70 % ethanol. The pellet was briefly air-dried and resuspended in aqua dest.

2.2. Medium scale preparation

For yielding higher amounts of plasmid DNA the medium scale preparation was used. A single bacterial colony was cultured in 2 ml TB-medium at 37 °C for five or six hours. Subsequently, the pre-culture was transferred to 100 ml TB-medium (plus appropriate antibiotic) and incubated at 37 °C in a shaker over night. Cells were harvested by centrifugation at 3300 rcf for 30 min at 4 °C.

Preparation

The 100 ml culture was transferred to two 50 ml tubes and centrifuged for 30 min at 3300 rcf and 4 °C. The cell pellet was resuspended in 3 ml Tris/EDTA/glucose solution by pipetting several times up and down. For cell lysis, 6 ml freshly made NaOH/SDS solution was added and incubated for 10 min at room temperature. Furthermore, 4.5 ml KAc was added, mixed by inverting the tube 6 times and incubated for 15 min on ice. The cell lysate was centrifuged for 20 min at 4 °C and 3300 rcf. The clear supernatant was transferred to a fresh 50 ml tube.

Precipitation

For a first precipitation step, twice the volume of ethanol was added to the supernatant, vortexed and additionally centrifuged at 3300 rcf for 30 min at 20 °C. The pellet was dried, resolved in 440 μl TE solution and transferred to a 1.5 ml tube.

220 μl 7.5 M ammonium acetate was added, vortexed and incubated for 20 min on ice. Subsequently, the sample was centrifuged for 15 min at 13000 rcf and 4 °C. The supernatant was transferred to a 2 ml tube and 1320 μl ethanol was added. For better precipitation the DNA/ethanol mixture was frozen for 1 hour at −80 °C and then centrifuged for 30 min at 13000 rcf and 4 °C. The washed and dried pellet was resolved in 200 μl TE solution.

RNA and protein degradation

For RNA degradation 2 μl 5 M NaCl and 5 μl RNase A solution (10 μg/μl) were added and incubated for 30 min at 37 C. For degradation of proteins, 2 μl 20 % SDS solution and 2 μl Proteinase K-solution were added and incubated for 30 min at 37 °C.

The DNA was further purified by phenol extraction and ethanol precipitation as described in Methods, chapter 5.1. Purification.

2.3. PAC and BAC plasmid isolation

Cells transfected with PAC and BAC vectors were specially treated because of the large size of the genomic DNA clone and the slow replication rate. The PAC vector (P1-derived artificial chromosome) is a plasmid of 16.5 kb containing a genomic insert of about 120 kb (Ioannou P et al. 1994). The PAC library was constructed by ligating a partial Sau3AI digest of human genomic DNA to the BamHI site of the PAC vector.

The BAC vector (Bacterial Artificial Chromosome) is a single copy plasmid holding an insert of about 120 kb size (Kim UJ et al. 1996). Ligating large size fractionated partial HindIII fragments to the HindIII site of the vector generated the BAC library. The human PAC library and a mouse BAC library were generated and screened by Genome Systems (St. Louis, Missouri) as described by (Erdel M et al. 1998, Meyer et al. 2000).

Cultivation of PAC carrying cells

A glycerol stock culture containing a PAC plasmid that carried the human SCYB11 sequence, was streaked out on LB-agar plates containing 25 µg/ml kanamycin. A colony was inoculated in 3.3 ml LB-broth containing less sodium chloride (preparation is described in Appendix, chapter 2. Solutions) supplemented with kanamycin and incubated over night at 37 °C in a shaker. The next day the preculture was transferred into 100 ml LB-broth with less sodium chloride plus kanamycin and shaken for 1.5 hours before 125 µl IPTG was added. (The PAC plasmid is maintained as a single copy per cell. IPTG, however, can increase the copy number by inducing the lytic operon.) The culture was further incubated for 5 hours. Bacteria were harvested by centrifugation at 9000 rcf for 30 min at 4 °C.

Cultivation of BAC carrying cells

A glycerol stock culture was streaked out on LB-agar plates containing 25 µg/ml chloramphenicol. A single colony was inoculated in 2 ml LB-broth and incubated in a shaker at 37 °C for 1 day. The preculture was transferred into 500 ml LB-broth (plus chloramphenicol) and incubated in a shaker over night. Next day, bacteria were harvested by centrifugation at 4500 rcf for 30 min at 4 °C.

Preparation of PAC and BAC plasmids

To isolate PAC and BAC plasmids from host cells, a *NUCLEOBOND® kit* was used with slight modifications in order to increase the DNA yield.

The bacterial culture was harvested by centrifugation at 3300 rcf for 30 min at 4 °C. Cells were resuspended in 5 ml *buffer S1* by pipetting the pellet several times up and down and transferred into a 50 ml tube. 5 ml *buffer S2* was added and gently mixed by inverting the tube 5 times. The mixture was incubated for 5 min at room temperature, before 5 ml *buffer S3* was added. The sample was mixed gently by inverting the tube 6 times. The mixture was incubated for 5 min on ice.

For clarification of the bacterial lysate, the mixture was centrifuged for a minimum of 2 hours at 3300 rcf at 4 °C. The supernatant was removed by filtration through a moistened folded filter into a new 50 ml tube.

Adsorption of DNA

The *Nucleobond AX cartridge* was equilibrated with 2 ml *buffer N2*. To bind the DNA, the lysate was loaded on the cartridge. After the equilibration-solution had moved through the cartridge, the bound DNA was washed twice with 4 ml *buffer N5*. Subsequently, plasmid DNA was eluted with 2 ml *buffer N5*.

Always, 1 ml of the collected eluate was transferred to a 2 ml tube and for precipitation, 700 µl isopropanol were added. The tubes were immediately centrifuged for 30 min at 13000 rcf and 4 °C and afterwards washed with 1 ml 70 % ethanol. For gentle resolving, 30 µl aqua dest were pipetted to the pellet and without vortexing the DNA was allowed to dissolve at 4 °C over night.

Dialysis

Solved DNA was pipetted on a 0.025 µm *Millipore filter* floating on a bath of sterile water in a petri dish and was dialysed for 2 hours.

Subsequently, ethanol precipitation was carried out as described in Methods, chapter 5.1.2. Ethanol precipitation.

2.4. Endotoxin-free plasmid isolation

For transfection of plasmid DNA into mammalian cells it is highly important to generate plasmid DNA of a very pure quality. For this purpose, we used the *Endo Free^{TM} Plasmid Maxi Kit* from Qiagen, which removes endotoxin (also known as LPS).

A single colony from a LB-Amp plate was picked and inoculated in 100 ml TB-medium supplemented with ampicillin. The culture was incubated for 18 h at 37 °C with vigorous shaking. For harvesting, the culture was divided into two 50 ml tubes and centrifuged for 30 min at 3300 rcf at 4 °C.

The two cell pellets were resuspended in 5 ml *P1 buffer* by pipetting the cells several times up and down. Subsequently 5 ml *P2 buffer* were added to each tube and mixed gently by inverting the tubes several times and, incubating them at room temperature for 5 min. Then 5 ml prechilled *P3 buffer* were added to each lysate and mixed by inverting gently for several times before both lysates were poured into the same barrel of the *QIAfilter cartridge*. The further procedure was carried according to the Qiagen handbook supplied with the kit.

The air dried pellet was resolved in 30 µl endotoxin free water. The yield of DNA was determined by UV spectrophotometry as described in Methods, <u>chapter 5.2. Optical density measurement.</u>

LAL-test

To determine the endotoxin content, a *Limulus amebocyte lysate* (LAL) test was performed. This test is a quantitative test for Gram-negative bacterial endotoxin. Briefly, the sample was mixed with the LAL supplied in the test kit and incubated at 37 °C for ten minutes. A substrate solution is then mixed with the LAL-sample and incubated at 37 °C for further six minutes. The reaction is stopped with stop reagent. If endotoxin is present in the sample, a yellow colour will develop. The absorbance of the sample can be determined specrophotometrically at 405-401 nm. Since this absorbance is in direct proportion to the amount of endotoxin present, the concentration of endotoxin can be calculated from a standard curve.

The DNA purified with the *Endotox free kit* contained only 13 EU/ml. This is just beyond the detection limit of the test (10 EU/ml), which is a neglectable amount for transfection.

3. Cell culture

3.1. Cell lines used

All cells were originally from the American Type culture collection ATCC; Rockville, MO, USA

- **THP-1 myelomonocytoma cells:** Cells were derived from the peripheral blood of a 1 year old male with acute monocytic leukemia. THP-1 cells grow in suspension in *RPMI 1640 medium* containing 10 % FCS and 2 mM L-glutamine.

- **RAW 264.7:** This monocyte-macrophage line was established from a tumour induced by Abelson Murine Leukemia Virus (A-MULV) in a male mouse. Cells were cultured in *X-VIVO 20 medium*. RAW264.7 cells are adherent and thus had to be scraped off the surface by a cell scraper.

- HepG2: Is a human hepatocellular carcinoma cell line. The line was derived from tissue of a 15-year-old male Caucasian. The cells are epithelial in morphology. This cell-line was used for transfection experiments as described in Methods, chapter 8.2. Cell transfection. The cells were cultured in *DMEM medium* containing 10 % FCS and 2 mM glutamine.

3.2. Culturing

Cells were cultured in an incubator providing them with an environment of 37 °C, 5 % CO_2, and almost 100 % humidity. The appropriate medium was buffered with a bicarbonate buffer system to keep the acid-base equilibrium stable. The 75 cm^2 culture flasks used, had a vent cap to allow gas exchange. The culture flasks were placed in the incubator in an upright position when cells were growing in suspension, whereas they were laid down for adherent growing.

For RNA isolation, 2.5×10^7 THP-1 myelomonocytoma cells were stimulated with 1250 U/ml human IFN-γ and 1 µg/ml LPS. The murine 2.5×10^7 RAW264.7 cells were stimulated with 250 U/ml murine IFN-γ plus 1 µg/ml LPS.

4. Isolation of genomic DNA and RNA of cultured cells

For all applications involving DNA and RNA sterile plastic ware and freshly autoclaved aqua dest was used. Moreover in all applications handling RNA, gloves had to be worn.

4.1. Isolation of genomic DNA

For cell lysis and preparation of genomic DNA the *"Qiagen Genomic DNA kit for blood, cultured cells, tissue, yeast and bacteria"* was used.

1×10^8 THP-1 myelomonocytoma cells were harvested by centrifugation for 10min at 1500 rcf and 4 °C and washed twice in 10 ml PBS. Cells were lysed following the lysis protocol for the maxi preparation of cell cultures. Subsequently, the protocol for genomic-tip 500/G volumes was followed. After eluting the genomic DNA in 15 ml buffer QF an additional phenol extraction step was carried out as described in Methods, chapter 5.1.1. Phenol extraction.

Subsequently, genomic DNA was precipitated with ethanol as described in Methods, chapter 5.1.2. Ethanol precipitation, and dissolved in aqua dest. For PCR applications, the genomic DNA was gently sheared by pipetting two or three times up and down.

4.2. Isolation of total RNA

2.5×10^7 cells were collected by centrifugation for 7 min at 1500 rcf at 20 °C. The supernatant was removed and the cell pellet was washed twice in 10 ml PBS. Subsequently cells were resuspended in 3 ml GTC buffer for lysis passed through a 20G-needle repetitively. At this stage, samples were either stored at -80 °C or the procedure was carried on immediately.

Acid Phenol Extraction

Total RNA was isolated by acid phenol extraction (Chomczynski P and Sacchi N. 1987) by mixing 3 ml *Rotiphenol* and 300 µl 2 M sodium acetate with the cell lysate. After rigorous vortexing, 750 µl chloroform/isoamyl alcohol was added, vortexed again and incubated for 15 min on ice. The mixture was centrifuged by 3300 rcf for 10 min at 4°C.

Precipitation

The aqueous phase was transferred into a RNase-free tube and mixed with 300 ml 3 M sodium acetate and 7.2 ml 100 % ethanol. For a better precipitation, tubes were incubated over night at -20 °C. The next day, total RNA was collected by centrifugation at 13000 rcf for 30 min at 4 °C. The supernatant was removed and the pellet was washed with 3 ml 70 % ethanol. After another centrifugation step, the pellet was briefly air-dried and then dissolved in 50 µl aqua dest. The concentration was determined by measuring the O.D. at 260 nm and 280 nm as described in Methods, chapter 5.2. Optical density measurement. Total RNA was stored at -80 °C.

4.3. Isolation of poly A$^+$ RNA

In general, 1 to 2 % of total RNA harvest from cell culture or tissue is poly-A$^+$ RNA. Poly A$^+$ RNA was isolated with the *Qiagen Oligotex^{TM} mRNA kit* following the protocol for oligotex spin column. The yield was determined by measuring the O.D. at $^{A260}/_{A280}$ nm as described in Methods, <u>chapter 5.2. Optical density measurement</u>.

5. Preparation and analysis of DNA and RNA

The methods listed below are written more generally as they were used very frequently and sometimes with small variations.

5.1. Purification

This chapter starts with the two mainly used purification methods since purity is required for all molecular biology techniques.

5.1.1. Phenol extraction

An equal volume of phenol/chloroform/isoamyl alcohol (25:24:1 V/V) was added to the same volume of DNA dissolved in aqua dest and vortexed vigorously. To separate the aqueous phase and the phenol phase, the mixture was centrifuged for 1 min at 13000 rcf at 20 °C. The aqueous phase (upper layer) containing the DNA was removed and transferred into a new 1.5 ml tube. The same volume chloroform/isoamyl alcohol (24:1 V/V) was added to the DNA solution and then vortexed again. The sample was centrifuged, and the aqueous phase (upper layer) was removed gently and transferred in a new tube. Afterwards, DNA was precipitated with ethanol as described below.

5.1.2. Ethanol precipitation

$^1/_{10}$ volume of 3 M sodium acetate (pH 5.2) was added to the solved DNA and vortexed. Further 2.5 volumes of 100 % ethanol was added and vortexed vigorously. For a better precipitation the mixture was either stored at -20 °C over night or at -80 °C for one hour.

DNA was collected by centrifugation at 13000 rcf for 30 min at 4 °C. The supernatant was removed and replaced by 1 ml 70 % ethanol. Subsequently, the sample was centrifuged for additional 10 min. Again more the supernatant was removed. The DNA pellet was air-dried, and dissolved in the appropriate volume of aqua dest.

5.2. Optical density measurement

DNA and RNA concentrations were calculated with the *KC4 Lambda Scan* (spectrophotometer for micro plate scanning). 1µl dissolved DNA was diluted in 500 µl aqua dest and UV absorbance was measured in a 96-well UV-plate at 260 nm. Factors used for calculation (50 for dsDNA and 40 for RNA) were multiplied with the absorbance value and the dilution factor 500. The purity of DNA / RNA was estimated from the ratio $^{A260}/_{A280}$ of the sample: pure DNA should have a ratio of 1.8, for RNA the ratio should be 2.0.

In addition, a pathlength correction for each well was carried out by measuring the absorbance at 977 nm and 900 nm. The formula for the pathlength correction is:

$$(A_{977} \text{ nm} - A_{900} \text{ nm}) \text{ well} \div (A_{977} \text{ nm} - A_{900} \text{ nm}) \times 1 \text{ cm water}.$$

The absorbance in the well is then divided by the pathlength.

5.3. Electrophoresis

In general, nucleic acids are negatively charged and migrate through the pores of an agarose gel to the positive lead. To separate DNA fragments of 100–10 000 bp in length, gels containing 1 % agarose were used.

5.3.1. Agarose gel electrophoresis

6 ml TBE 1x electrophoresis buffer (supplemented with ethidium bromide as described in the Appendix, chapter 2. Solutions) was mixed with 0.6 g agarose and

heated in a microwave oven until the agarose was dissolved. The mixture was poured into a gel casting platform with an inserted gel comb.

The cooled agarose gel was placed into an electrophoresis tank containing 1x TBE supplemented with ethidium bromide as running buffer. The DNA samples were prepared with the appropriate amount of 6x loading buffer and loaded into the wells. Electrophoresis was performed at 50 V for 1 hour or longer (depending on the size of DNA).

The DNA bands, stained with ethidium bromide, were visualized on a *UV transilluminator* and photographed with a *Polaroid type 667/ black and white instant film*.

5.3.2. Isolation of DNA restriction fragments from agarose gels

20 to 50 µg of plasmid DNA were digested with restriction enzymes as described in Methods, chapter 6.1. Digestion of DNA with restriction endonucleases. DNA bands were separated on TBE-agarose gel (see Methods, chapter 5.3.1. Agarose gel electrophoresis). DNA stained with ethidium bromide was visualized on a UV-transilluminator. After photographing, the appropriate DNA band was excised with a razor blade and transferred into a sterile 1.5 ml tube. DNA was isolated from the gel with the *Qiaquick Gel Extraction Kit* (Qiagen).

The procedure was carried according to the manufactories protocol *using a microcentrifuge*. 1 to 5 µl of eluated DNA were loaded on a TBE agarose gel supplemented with ethidium bromide. To estimate the DNA concentration, the fluorescence intensity of the purified DNA fragment and the marker were compared.

5.3.3. Formaldehyde gel electrophoresis

2 g agarose was dissolved in 144 ml aqua dest and heated in a microwave before 20 ml 10x MOPS was added. When the mixture had cooled to 50 °C, 36 ml formaldehyde was added and the gel was poured into a gel casting plat form with a gel comb inserted. Prior to use, the comb was removed and the gel was submersed

into a horizontal electrophoreses chamber containing 1x MOPS running buffer supplemented with ethidium bromide.

For RNA sample preparation, 15 µl of the RNA loading mix (listed in the Appendix, chapter 2. Solutions) was added to 10 µg of total RNA. The sample was topped up with aqua dest to a final volume of 20 µl. The sample was incubated for 10 min at 56 °C in a water bath and subsequently placed on ice. 2 µl loading buffer was added and the RNA sample was loaded into the wells. The gel was run at 50 V for 3.5 hours to let RNA migrate to the positive lead.

18 S and 28 S RNA bands stained with ethidium bromide was visualized on the *UV-transilluminator* and photographed with a *Polaroid type 667/ black and white instant film*.

5.4. Southern blot / Northern blot

Blotting is a technique in which nucleic acid fragments are transferred from a gel to a nylon or nitrocellulose membrane. For this work a *Duralon-UV* nylon membrane (Stratagene) was used. Nucleic acids were fixed to the membrane by UV-light using a *Stratalinker*. After blotting the fragment of interest were identified by hybridization with a labelled DNA probe.

The procedure for Northern blot (transfer of RNA to a membrane) and for Southern blot (transfer of DNA to a membrane) is identical. The only difference is that DNA has to be denatured before blotting.

Denaturation of DNA

DNA was denatured by soaking the gel into a denaturation solution for 30 min (see Appendix, chapter 2. Solutions). After 15 min, the denaturation solution was replaced by a fresh solution. Subsequently, the gel was soaked in a neutralization solution for additional 30 min.

Vacuum-blotting

A sheet of *Whatman filter paper* and a *Duralon-UV membrane* were moisten in aqua dest. Filter paper, nylon membrane and the gel were placed on the *Vacu-Blotter-System*. Blotting was performed at 0.2 bar for 2 hours. During blotting the gel was kept wet by repetitively adding 20x SSC.

Finally, the gel wells were marked on the membrane with a pencil. After the gel was removed, the membrane was shortly washed in aqua dest to remove any agarose gel residues. Fixation of RNA on the membrane was achieved by UV radiation lasting 30 sec in a *UV Stratalinker*. The fixed membrane was air-dried and wrapped in saran food-wrap until the following day.

5.5. Hybridization analysis of blots with radiolabelled DNA probes

The principle of hybridization is that a single-stranded DNA (called probe) can hybridize to a complementary DNA or RNA fixed on a nylon membrane. The probe is a DNA fragment of 100 to 500 bp length which was labelled with α^{32}-P.

5.5.1. List of probes

The probes were mainly generated by PCR. Primer sequences are listed in Methods, chapter 7.1.2. List of primers.

Human
- **mg** is a 268 bp genomic sequence and comprises exon 2, intron 2, and exon 3, of SCYB11 genomic DNA. The probe was amplified by PCR using the primer pair migbse1.prim and migbse2.prim.
- **Mig-b ges** is a 730 bp cDNA sequence and was isolated by Xbal endonuclease digestion of the human CXCL11 cDNA clone. The probe comprises a part of exon 4 beginning behind the stop codon.

- **huSCYBINT1** was amplified with the primer pair huSCYBint1.prim and huSCYBint2.prim from human PAC 17352. The probe is 270 bp long and hybridises to intron 1 of human SCYB11.

Murine

- **mumig** is a PCR product amplified with the primer pair mumig1.prim and mumig2.prim from genomic DNA isolated from RAW264.7 cells and is 215 bp long. It hybridises to exon 2, intron 2, and exon 3.

The purified probes were stored at -20 °C until usage.

5.5.2. Radiolabelling of probes

α-Labelled CTP^{32} is a deoxycytidine triphosphate where the innermost phosphor atom is radioactive labelled.

The following reaction mix was prepared in a sterile 1.5 ml tube:

    18 µl aqua dest.

    1 µl random hexamer primers

    2 µl purified DNA probe

DNA was denatured for 5 min in a 95 °C water bath and subsequently placed on ice to let the random hexamer primers bind to DNA. Subsequently it was added:

    3 µl Klenow fragment buffer 10x

    4 µl α^{32}-P dCTP

    1 µl Klenow fragment

    The elongation reaction was incubated for 1 hour at 37 °C in a water bath.

Purification of radiolabelled probes

To separate labelled DNA from unincorporated radioactive precursor, the *Qiagen Qiaquick Nucleotide Removal Kit* (for microcentrifuge) was used. The DNA was eluted in 30 ml aqua dest. Just before hybridization the probes were denatured by heating in a 95 °C water bath for 5 min and subsequently placed on ice.

Measuring radioactivity

To confirm a successful integration of α^{32}-P, 1 µl of the eluted probe was mixed with 2 ml scintillation fluid in a scintillation vial. The cpm was measured in a *liquid scintillation counter* for 30 sec. To calculate the dilution, counts were multiplied by the dilution-factor 30. In case of a successful integration the cpm should be 3×10^7 or more.

5.5.3. Hybridization of DNA blots

The hybridization solution for Southern blots was made freshly before use. The same solution was used for prehybridization and hybridization.

The nylon membrane carrying the immobilized DNA was soaked in 1x SSC. The membrane was placed in a hybridization tube (DNA facing inside) and 12 ml hybridization solution was added.

For pre-hybridization, the membrane was incubated in an hybridization oven with rotation for 3 to 4 hours at 42 °C. Towards the end of the prehybridization time, the appropriate probe was radioactively labelled as described in Methods, chapter 5.5.2. Radiolabelling of probes. The solution for prehybridization was replaced by an equal amount of hybridization solution and the labelled probe was added.

The membrane was further incubated over night under the same conditions. The next day, the hybridization solution was replaced by 20 ml 2x SSPE + 0.5 % SDS and further incubated for 30 min in the hybridization oven.

Thereafter, the solution was exchanged by a more stringent wash solution (1x SSPE + 0.5 % SDS) and once more incubated for 30 min in the oven. For a high-stringency wash, the blot was additionally washed twice with 0.1x SSPE + 0.1 % SDS at 50 °C.

After the final washing step, the membrane was wrapped in *Saran food Wrap* and autoradiographed using *Kodak X-OMAT* X-ray films and intensifying screens at -80 °C.

5.5.4. Hybridization of RNA blots

The hybridization solution for Northern blots (see Appendix, <u>chapter 2. Solutions</u>) was always made freshly before used. To avoid background, sodium pyrophosphate and dextran should be solved very carefully.

The nylon membrane carrying immobilized RNA was soaked with 1x SSC before placing it into the hybridization tube (RNA side up).

For prehybridization, the RNA was incubated with 12 ml hybridization solution for 3 or 4 hours at 65 °C in a hybridization oven with rotations. The probe was labelled just before the end of the prehybridization time. Afterwards, the prehybridization solution was exchanged by 12 ml fresh hybridization solution mixed with radiolabelled probe. Hybridization was continued over night at 65 °C.

Washing

Hybridization solution was replaced by 20 ml 2x SSC + 0.5 % SDS. After 30 min, the wash solution was exchanged against the more stringent 1x SSC + 0.5 % SDS wash solution. For a high stringency wash, the membrane was spreaded out in a plastic dish filled with 500 ml 0.1x SSC + 0.1 % SDS washing solution and incubated for 30 min in a 50 °C water-bath. After the final washing step, excess fluid was wiped off the membrane, which was then covered in *Saran food wrap*, for analysis.

Analysis

The *storage phosphorimager phosphor screen* was exposed to light for 20 min, to totally clear the screen. The membrane was fixed to the inside of the exposure cassette and the screen was placed on top of the membrane. The screen was exposed to the radioactively labelled blot up to four days.

Thereafter, the screen was scanned with the *Storm 840 scanner* and the signal was analysed, using the *Image Quant software*.

5.6. Fibre FISH experiments (List of probes)

To identify the position of probes on metaphase chromosomes, FISH (fluorescent *in situ* hybridization) is a widely used technique. Fibre FISH is a recently developed method working with stretched duplex DNA fibres. This technique is helpful in resolving gene arrangement by mapping their locations. The sensitivity of fibre FISH is such that typically probes of 1 kb can be detected on DNA fibres.

In our approach, PCR fragments of different sizes derived from exon and intron sequences were hybridised together with the complete PAC / BAC clone on an extended DNA fibre. The DNA fibres were derived from cultured cells. The result is a multi-colour image in which the arrangement of DNA probes along an extended strand of DNA is observed (Parra I and Windle B 1993).

The probes were labelled with fluorescent dyes and hybridizations were evaluated using a fluorescence microscope. Preparation of DNA fibres and hybridization with labelled probes and evaluation was performed in the Department of Medical Biology by Martin Erdel and colleagues.

Probes for human SCYB11, SCYB10 and SCYB9

All primers are listed in Methods, chapter 7.1.2. List of primers.

* **HuSCYB11** probe is 3.5 kb long. The sequence is derived from PAC 17352 digested with XbaI. The restriction fragment was subcloned into the *Blueskript SK⁻ vector*. The sequence comprises a part of exon 4 behind the stop codon and the surrounding DNA.

- **IP-10S** is 3000 bp in length and was generated with primer pair IP-10gen.prim and IP-10 genR.prim from PAC 17352. The probe comprises a part of the promoter region, and exon 1 to the stop codon within exon 4.
- **MigS** is 5200 bp and was generated with primer pair famiggen.prim and famiggeR.prim from PAC 17532 and hybridises to exon 1 to exon 4.

Probes for murine *Scyb11*, *Scyb10* and *Scyb9*

- **muscyb11** generated with primer pair muscyb11ex1.prim and muscybex4r.prim from BAC 22256 is 3000 bp long. The probe comprises exon 1 to exon 4, including start and stop codon.
- **muIP-10** is a PCR product of BAC 22256, amplified with primer pair muIP-10-2.prim and muIP-10-3.prim and is 3000 bp long. The sequence comprises about 1500 bp of the promoter region and exon 1 to exon 4.
- **mufaMIG** is 4.1 kb in size and was amplified with mumigfar1.prim and mumigfar2.prim. The probe hybridises to a region spanning exon 1 to exon 4.

6. Enzymatic manipulation of DNA and RNA

6.1. Digestion of DNA with restriction endonucleases

Restriction endonucleases are enzymes that cleave double-stranded DNA at specific sites. Enzyme activity is defined in units: one unit is the amount of restriction endonucleases needed to completely digest 1 µg of purified DNA in 60 min.

All restriction endonucleases were obtained from Promega. For a single restriction endonuclease digestion, 10x buffer supplied with each restriction enzyme was used. For multiple restriction digestion the optimal buffer was chosen from a *list of relative activity of restriction enzyme in Promega buffer*.

Digestion of 1 µg DNA

  1 µg DNA

  aqua dest to bring volume to 8 µl

  1 µl appropriate 10x restriction buffer

  1 µl restriction endonuclease

The reaction mixture was vortexed and incubated for 1 hour at the recommended temperature (in general 37 °C). After digestion, the DNA fragments obtained from digestion were separated on agarose gels and the DNA bands were visualized under UV-light as described in Methods, chapter 5.3.1. Agarose gel electrophoresis.

6.2. Ligation

Ligation is an enzymatic reaction to join a vector and a specific DNA fragment with homologous cohesive ends. In principle, a DNA ligase catalyses the formation of phosphodiester bonds between a juxtaposed 5′-phosphate and a 3′-hydroxyl terminus.

6.2.1. Subcloning of DNA fragments into the pBluescript SK⁻ vector

Preparation of vector and insert

DNA fragments were obtained by restriction endonuclease cleavage. The digested DNA was separated on an agarose gel and the desired band was cut out and removed from the gel with the *Qiagen Gel Extraction Kit* (Qiagen).

The vector was digested with the same endonucleases in order to create homologous cohesive ends. The linearized vector was dephosphorilated by adding 2 µl *calf intestine alkaline phosphatase* and incubated at 37 °C for 30 min.

The vector was purified by separation on an agarose gel and extracted using the *Qiaquick Gel Extraction Kit*. After ethanol precipitation, the vector DNA was resuspended in the same volume of aqua dest as the insert DNA.

Ligation

To estimate the amount of vector and insert DNA, 1 µl of each sample was separated by agarose gel electrophoresis. For ligation, the ideal ratio of insert to vector DNA is variable. Usually three or four different ligation mixes with variable concentration and ratio were set up.

Vector DNA (1 - 4 µl) and insert DNA (1 - 4 µl) were mixed with 1 µl ligase-buffer. The volume was brought with aqua dest to 9.2 µl before 0.8 µl T4 ligase was added. This ligation reaction was incubated at 12 °C over night using a *thermal cycler* (Perkin Elmer).

The next day, a total volume of 10 µl of the ligation reaction was added to the calcium chloride-treated competent bacteria and transformation was carried out as described in Methods, chapter 1.3. Transformation with calcium chloride.

6.2.2. Ligation into TA-vector

Taq-polymerase has a non-template depending activity adding a single adenosine to the 3´ end of PCR-products. This A-overhang can be used for cloning, thus TA-vectors have a single 3´ thymidine overhang. In addition, the *TOPO-TA-vector* has a covalently bound topoisomerase, which provides a very efficient and fast cloning reaction.

The cloning reaction was carried out as described in the TOPO^{TM} TA Cloning-Instruction manual (Invitrogen). Immediately after cloning, transformation was carried out as described in the manual, using *TOPO 10F cells* supplied with the kit.

6.2.3. Ligation into pGL3$_{basis}$ vector

The pGL3 vector is a reporter vector, which contains a reporter gene (firefly luciferase gene) but no promoter. A part of the human SCYB11 promoter was inserted upstream of the reporter gene. After insertion of the promoter, the promoter elements could regulate the expression of luciferase activity in mammalian cells transfected with the vector-construct.

Insertion of MluI and BglII restriction cleavage sites into the CXCL11 promoter

A 3500 bp fragment of human SCYB11 promoter was isolated from PAC 17352 by digestion with HindIII. This promoter sequence was further amplified with two primers carrying specific mutations. The PCR product was subcloned into *TA-Cloning vector* for propagation.

hupromB.prim	sense	GAAGCTTATCGAACGCGTCAACTCATC
hupromM.prim	anti-sense	GCTTTGCAGATCTTCTTGGAAGGAGTAG

The primer hpromM.prim contains three single nucleotide exchanges to create a MluI restriction cleavage site. The hupromB.prim contains two single nucleotide exchanges to create a BglII cleavage site.

Ligation of the SCYB11 promoter into the pGL3$_{basis}$ vector

The pGL3$_{basis}$ vector was digested with BglII and MluI restriction enzymes. Subsequently, vector DNA was treated with calf intestinal alkaline phosphatase to remove the 5´ phosphate groups. (This decreased the background of non-recombinants.) To prepare compatible ends, human promoter fragments were digested with the same restriction enzymes.

Both linearized vector and insert DNA were purified by electrophoresis on an agarose gel and then recovered by the *Qiaquick Gel Extraction Kit* (Qiagen). To estimate the ratio of vector to insert, equal amounts of linearized vector and purified insert were loaded on an agarose gel.

Vector DNA (1-3 µl) and insert DNA (1-2 µl) were mixed with 1 µl ligase buffer and 0.8 µl T4 DNA ligase and brought to a total volume of 10 µl with aqua dest. The ligation reaction was incubated at 12 °C over night using a *thermal cycler* (Perkin Elmer).

Calcium chloride competent XL-1 cells were used for transformation. Transformation was carried out as described in Methods, chapter 1.3. Transformation with calcium chloride.

6.2.4. Cloning into pET32-a expression vector

The *pET-32a* is a vector for expression of recombinant protein in *E.coli*. The polypeptide sequence is fused with a histidine Tag (His-Tag), which facilitates protein purification, and a thioredoxin fusion tag (Trx-Tag). The thioredoxin fusion tag enhances the solubility of target protein and catalyses the formation of disulfide bonds.

Restriction digestion of vector and insert

The open reading frame of human SCYB11 promoter was cut with the restriction endonuclease XhoI and KpnI from the TA-vector. To create cohesive ends, *pET-32a vector* was also digested with XhoI and KpnI. The vector was dephosphorylated with calf intestinal alkaline phosphatase.

The DNA fragments of vector and insert were purified by agarose gel electrophoresis and purified using the *Qiagen Gel-extraction kit*.

Vector and insert were ligated with T4 DNA ligase at 12 °C over night as outlined above. The plasmid was transformed into competent XL-1 as described in Methods, chapter 1.3. Transformation with calcium chloride.

6.3. Reverse Transcription

Reverse transcriptase is an enzyme that generates DNA copies from RNA to synthesize complementary DNA (cDNA).

Total RNA was precipitated in 100 % ethanol and washed in 70 % ethanol. The RNA pellet was gently air-dried and subsequently dissolved in an appropriate volume of aqua dest. 1 µl of the solved RNA was taken for optical density measurement. To ensure complete reverse transcription, not more than 1 µg of total RNA was used for the enzymatic reaction:

> x µl aqua dest to bring the volume to 50 µl
>
> 10 µl 5x first strand buffer
>
> 5 µl dNTPs (10 mM)
>
> 5 µl DTT 0,1 M
>
> 2 µl oligo-dT primers (1 µg/µl)
>
> 2 µl RNase inhibitor
>
> 1 µg total RNA
>
> 2 µl Superscript II RT (200 U/µl)

RNasin, RNA and Reverse Transcriptase were added after all the other reagents had been mixed on ice.

6.4. Unidirectional digestion with exonuclease III

This method fulfils a unidirectional digestion of an insert DNA without any further subcloning. Exonuclease III has the specific enzyme activity to digest only DNA from a 5´ protruding or blunt end. The specific assay of DNA linearization, unidirectional digestion with exonuclase III and subsequent religation was first described by (Henikoff S 1987). This strategy was used to create human SCYB11 promoter fragments of different size.

Exonuclease III digestion

Human SCYB11 promoter fragment was cloned into the reporter vector pGL3$_{basis}$. To create a 5´overhang, the plasmid was digested with MluI. To protect the 3´ end from endonuclease III it was cut with KpnI thus creating a 3´ protrusion. DNA was purified with phenol extraction and ethanol precipitation.

The pellet was dissolved in 60 µl Exo-buffer and warmed up to 37 °C before 2.5 µl exonuclease III was added. The sample was mixed well before continuing to incubate at 37 °C. Every 30 sec, 2.5 µl were removed from the exonuclease digestion reaction into an appropriate tube containing 7.5 µl S1 mix. The tubes were kept on ice until all aliquots were removed.

Subsequently, the S1 digestion was stopped by adding 1 µl of S1 stop solution and heating up to 70 °C for 10 min. To visualize the actual extent of digestion, 2 µl of each sample was removed and loaded onto an agarose gel. Selected aliquots were precipitated with ethanol in presence of sodium acetate. The dried DNA pellets were solved in 9 µl TE-buffer.

Religation

1 µl Klenow buffer and 0.5 µl Klenow fragment were added to the DNA dissolved in TE buffer and incubated for 3 min at 37 °C. Then, 1 µl 0.125 mM dNTP mix were supplied and continued to incubate at 37 °C for 5 min.

Subsequently, the Klenow fragment was heat-inactivated for 10 min at 65 °C. In a final step, 40 µl T4-ligase mix was added to each aliquot and this was incubated for 1.5 hours at room temperature. The religated plasmids were then transformed into competent XL-1 cells, which were then cultivated on LB-agar plates supplemented with ampicillin.

6.5. Site-directed mutagenesis

The human SCYB11 cDNA (cloned in *pET-32a expression vector*) was missing the first amino acid phenylalanine. Therefore, the nucleotide triplet TTC coding for the amino acid phenylalanine was inserted with the *Quick Change site-directed mutagenesis kit* (Stratagene). In this procedure, a double stranded DNA vector gets completely copied with DNA polymerase using two oligonucleotide primers containing the desired mutation.

The primers (Microsynth) were designed to be complementary to opposite strands of the vector and contained the mutation in the middle (bold letters). The following formula was used to estimate the T_m of the primers:

$$Tm = 81.5 + 0.41 \, (\% \, GC) - 675 \, / \, N - \% \, \text{mismatches}$$

migfins1.prim	sense	CCGACGACGACGACAAG**TTC**CCCATGTTC AAAAGAGGACG
migfins2.prim	complementary	CGTCCTCTTTTGAACATGGG**GAA**CTTGTCG TCGTCGTCGG

The reaction mixture was prepared as follows using the *Quick Change kit* (Stratagene):

> 5 µl 10x reaction buffer
>
> 12.5 µg of pET32-a vector
>
> 1.25 µl primer migfins1 (8.8 mM)
>
> 1.25 µl primer migfins2 (8.8 mM)
>
> 1 ml dNTP mix
>
> aqua dest to a final volume of 50 µl
>
> 1 µl of Pfu Turbo DNA polymerase (2.5 U/µl)

Cycling parameters:

1 cycle:	30 sec 95 °C
16 cycles:	30 sec 95 °C
	1 min 55 °C
	12 min 68 °C

Following temperature cycling, the reaction was cooled to 37 °C. 1 µl of DpnI restriction enzyme was added directly to the amplification reaction to digest the parental (non-mutated) DNA strands. The reaction was continued to incubate at 37 °C for 1 hour.

The plasmid containing the desired mutation was transformed into competent XL-1 cells. The cells were spreaded on LB-agar plates supplemented with ampicillin.

6.6. Primer extension

Primer extension is used to map the 5′ terminus of RNA. The technique utilizes reverse transcriptase to extend a primer that is complementary to a certain region of the RNA. Total RNA was isolated from THP-1 cells stimulated with 1250 U/ml IFN-γ and 1 µg LPS as described in Methods, chapter 4.2. Isolation of total RNA.

6.6.1. Endlabelling of the primer

migtrans.prim	anti-sense	TGGTGCTGTTGCTGCTACTTCAGC

The following reagents were mixed in the order indicated:

3.5 µl aqua dest.

1 µl 10x kinase buffer

1 µl 1 mM spermidine

1 µl primer migtrans.prim (10 µM)

3 µl P-γ^{32} ATP

0.5 µl T4 polynucleotide kinase

The reaction was incubated for 1 hour at 37 °C. To stop the activity of T4 kinase, 2 µl 0,5 M EDTA and 50 µl TE buffer were added and heated to 65 °C for 5 min.

6.6.2. Purification of the primer

The primer was purified with *NICK® Spin columns*. The columns are designed for separation of DNA fragments from γ^{32}-P labelled nucleotides. The procedure was carried out as described in the instruction manual. For equilibration, TE buffer + 600 mM NaCl was used.

The labelling of γ^{32}-P (dATP) was measured as described in Methods, <u>chapter 5.5.2. Radiolabelling of probes</u>.

6.6.3. Hybridization and Primer extension

The following was mixed in a 1.5 ml tube:

> 10 µl (14.7 µg) poly A$^+$ RNA
>
> 1,5 µl 10x hybridization buffer
>
> 3.5 µl radiolabelled primer

The mix was incubated at 67 °C (7 °C below the calculated annealing temperature) in a water bath. After 30 min the water bath was turned off to allow the tube to cool down slowly and to let the primer anneal to the RNA.

The following primer extension mix was prepared in a 1.5 ml tube:

> 0.9 µl 0.1M TrisCl (pH 8.3)
>
> 0.9 µl 0.5 M MgCl$_2$
>
> 0.25 µl 1 M DTT
>
> 6.75 µl 1 mg/ml actinomycin D
>
> 1.33 µl 5 mM dNTP mix (10 mM)
>
> 20 µl aqua dest.
>
> 0.5 µl Superscript II RT

30 µl of this mix was added to the tube containing the RNA. The mix incubated for 1 hour at 42 °C.

6.6.4. RNase digestion and purification

After cDNA amplification 5 µl RNase A was added to the tube containing the reaction mix and incubated for 15 min at 37 °C. When all RNA was completely digested, the cDNA was phenol purified and ethanol precipitated as described in

Methods, <u>chapter 5.1. Purification</u>. The dried pellet was resuspended in 5 µl loading buffer and heated for 5 min in a 65 °C water bath.

The sample was loaded on a polyacrylamide sequencing gel and separated together with a sequencing reaction (described in Methods, <u>chapter 6.7. DNA Sequencing</u>) at 1500 V for 1 hour.

6.7. DNA Sequencing

The DNA sequencing technique (Sanger method) is based on generation of short DNA sequences in four separate enzymatic reactions, where all oligonucleotides terminate at variable ends of A, T, G, C. In this enzymatic sequencing method, a DNA polymerase is utilized to synthesize a labelled, complementary copy of a DNA template. When a ddNMP is incorporated at the 3´end of the growing chain, chain elongation is terminated because the primer chain now lacks a 3´-hydroxyl group. The oligonucleotide products of the four reactions are resolved on adjacent lanes of a sequencing gel. For electrophoresis procedures, a high-resolution denaturing polyacrylamide gel was used, which is capable of resolving single-stranded oligonucleotides which differ in size by a single nucleotide.

6.7.1. Labelling and termination of the sequencing reaction

For the thermal cycle sequence reaction, the *Delta Tth Polymerase Sequencing Kit* (Clontech) was used. The procedure was carried out as described in the manual supplied with the kit.

In each of the four PCR tubes, which were placed on ice, 2 µl ddATP, 2 µl ddCTP, 2 µl ddGTP or 2 µl ddTTP were pipetted.

The following reagents were mixed in a 1.5 ml tube:

> 6 µg template DNA
>
> (with aqua dest diluted to a final volume of 102 µl)

3 µl reaction buffer

1 µl primer (10 µM)

0.8 µl dNTP mix

1 µl α-^{32}P-dATP

1 µl T4 polymerase

4 µl of the reaction mix was added to the PCR tubes containing 2 µl ddATP, ddCTP, ddGTP or ddTTP. The tubes were placed in the thermal cycler (*Gene Amp PCR System* / Perkin Elmer).

The following PCR conditions were used:

1 cycle:	5 min at 95 °C
30 cycles:	30 sec at 95 °C
	120 sec at 72 °C

subsequently cooled down to 4 °C

To terminate the reaction, 4 µl stop-solution was added to each tube. The reaction was stored at -20 °C over night.

6.7.2. Sequencing gel

A pair of 37 x 40 cm glass plates was washed with ethanol and subsequently with aqua dest. After drying a film of *Sigmacote* was applied on one of the glass plates and wiped dry. The gel plates were assembled with 4 mm spacers.

The gel was mixed as follows:

100 ml polyacrylamide urea solution

1 ml 10 % ammonium persulfate

40 µl TEMED

The gel was poured immediately after mixing. Afterwards, a *shark toothcomb* was inserted.

The gel was prewarmed for 45 min at 1500 V before 4 µl of each sequencing sample was loaded per well. The gel was electophoresed for 3 hours and 30 min at 60 W. The warm gel was removed from the glass plates, spreaded on *Whatman-chromatograpy paper* and covered with *saran foil*. The gel was dried at 80 °C in a gel dryer and subsequently placed into an X-ray cassette and autoradiographed at room temperature over night.

7. Polymerase Chain Reaction

Polymerase Chain Reaction (PCR) is a rapid procedure to amplify a specific segment of DNA. This method was used for various applications including direct cloning from genomic DNA or cDNA and detection of sequence variations and to generate probes for hybridization experiments.

In general all PCR reactions were pipetted with sterile filter tips (listed in Appendix, chapter 5. Materials). All primers used were synthesized by Microsynth GmbH (Switzerland).

7.1. Taq polymerase

7.1.1.Use of Taq antibody

This antibody (*TaqStart Antibody* / Clontech) binds to and inactivates DNA polymerase of Thermus aquaticus. Therefore the antibody is used to block polymerase activity during set-up of the PCR reaction at room temperature. At the first template denaturation step in thermal cycling the enzyme-antibody complex dissociates and the activity of Taq DNA polymerase is completely restored.

Preparation of Taq antibody- Taq polymerase complex

The concentrated *TaqStart^{TM}* Antibody (Clontech) was added directly to the equal volume of Taq polymerase. The mixture was incubated at room temperature for 5 min to allow for antibody binding. For storage, the mixture was aliqoted and kept frozen at -20 °C until usage.

7.1.2. List of primers

The primers were sent as lyophilized DNA pellets. The DNA was dissolved in 1ml TE buffer (see Appendix, chapter 2. Solutions) and incubated for 5 min at 50 °C. The primers were generally diluted to a concentration of 10 µM.

Primers for human CXCL11

migbse1.prim	forward	GAGGACGCTGTCTTTGCATAGGC
huscyb11gen2.prim	reverse	GTCAATGTCTCCACCGTAACCAC

To isolate the missing part of the genomic sequence (part of exon 4) of human SCYB11 from PAC 17352.

migbse2.prim	reverse	AGCCTTGCTTGCTTCGATTTGGG

Together with migbse1.prim this primer was taken to isolate a genomic fragment of human SCYB11. The PCR product was used as a probe for Southern blots. See also Methods, chapter 5.5.1. List of probes.

huSCYBint1.prim	forward	GCGATCATGTTAACAAGCTTCCTG
huSCYBint2.prim	reverse	CTGATTGCAACAGATGGCTGTGG

These primers were designed to amplify intron 1 of the human SCYB11 gene from PAC 17352. The sequence was used as a probe to detect unspliced mRNA (pre mRNA) on Northern blots. See also Methods, chapter 5.5.1. List of probes.

hpromM.prim	forward	CAAGCTTATCGAACGCGTCAACTCATC
hpromB.prim	reverse	GCTTTGCAGATCTTCTTGGAAGGAGTAG

Primers carrying a MluI (hpromM.prim) and a BgI II (hpromB.prim) restriction cleavage site were designed to amplify the human SCYB11 promoter, which was cloned into the pGL3$_{basis}$ vector. See also Methods, <u>chapter 6.2.3. Ligation into pGL3$_{basis}$ vector</u>.

Primers for human CXCL9 and CXCL10

hip10ex1.prim	forward	GCGATTCTGATTTGCTGCCTTATC
hip10ex2.prim	reverse	CTAATGCTGATGCAGGTACAGCG
hfamigex1.prim	forward	CATCATCTTGCTGGTTCTGATTGG
hfamigex2.prim	reverse	GTTGGTGCTGATGCAGGAACAGC

These primers were designed to detect and isolate the genomic sequence of SCYB9 and SCYB10 on the human PAC 17532 clone.

ip10gene.prim	forward	TGATCAAGGAGGACTGTCCAGG
ip10genR.prim	reverse	CAACCAAGTGACACACAAGGCAC
famiggen.prim	forward	CAGGAGTGACTTGGAACTCCATTC
famiggeR.prim	reverse	CACCTGCTCTGAGACAATGGTC

Primers were designed to amplify a ~3000 bp fragment of the genomic sequence SCYB10 and a ~4000 bp fragment of SCYB9 from human PAC 17352 clone. These PCR products were used as probes for fibre-FISH experiments. See also Methods, <u>chapter 5.6. Fibre FISH experiments and list of probes</u>.

Primers for murine CXCL11

| migbse1.prim | forward | GAGGACGCTGTCTTTGCATAGGC |
| migbse2.prim | reverse | AGCCTTGCTTGCTTCGATTTGGG |

The primers were designed from consensus regions of the human CXCL11 cDNA sequence. With this primer pair, the first isolation of a murine CXCL11 cDNA fragment was obtained. As a template, total RNA isolated from RAW264.7 cells stimulated with 250 U/ml murine IFN-γ and 1 µg LPS for 7 hours, was taken. See also Methods, <u>chapter 5.5.1. List of probes.</u>

mumig1	forward	GGATGAAAGCCGTCAAAATGGC
mumig2	reverse	GGTCCAGGCACCTTTGTCG

This primer pair was used to generate a genomic fragment of murine *Scyb11*. The genomic DNA used as template was isolated from unstimulated RAW264.7 cells. The fragment was used as a probe for Southern blots. See also Methods, <u>chapter 5.5.1. List of probes.</u>

muscyb11ex1.prim	forward	CGTTGCTCTCTGCAAAGAGAGATC
muscyb11ex2.prim	reverse	CAACTTTGTCGCAGCCGTTACTC

Primers were designed to amplify intron 1 of murine *Scyb11* from the murine BAC 22256 clone.

Primers for murine *Scyb9* and *Scyb10*

muip10-1.prim	forward	CTGCCTCATCCTGCTGGGTC
muip10-2.prim	reverse	GCTTCTCTCCAGTTAAGGAGC
mumigfar1.prim	forward	GGCATCATCTTCCTGGAGCAC
mumigfar2.prim	reverse	GTCTTCCTTGAACGACGACGAC

Primers were designed to obtain genomic sequence parts of murine *Scyb10* and *Scyb9* respectively, which are also located on the murine BAC 22256 clone.

muscyb11ex1.prim	forward	CGTTGCTCTCTGCAAAGAGAGATC
muscybex4r.prim	reverse	CCTGTACGTCTGGTTTTATCAGTG
muIP10-3.prim	forward	GATCTGCTCTTTGGAGACACTG

Primers were designed to amplify genomic DNA sequences of about 3000 kb as probes for fibre-FISH experiment. As an antisense primer for muIP-10.prim, the former primer muIP10-2.prim was used. See also Methods, <u>chapter 5.6. Fibre FISH experiments (list of probes)</u>.

7.1.3. Standard procedure for PCR amplification

For most applications, Taq Polymerase (Promega) was used. The common feature of Taq polymerase is a $5'\rightarrow3'$ DNA polymerase activity and a $5'\rightarrow3'$ exonuclease activity.

Furthermore, Taq polymerase has a non template-dependent terminal transferase activity that adds a single desoxyadenosine (A) to the $3'$end of PCR products. This feature was used to clone PCR fragments into TA vectors. See also Methods, <u>chapter 6.2.2. Ligation into TA-vector</u>.

PCR amplification

The reaction mix was set up at room temperature.

In a sterile nuclease-free PCR-tube, the following components were added:

> 4 µl $MgCl_2$ (25 mM)
>
> 5 µl 2 mM NTP mix
>
> 5 µl thermophilic DNA Polymerase 10x buffer (magnesium free)
>
> 1 µl 20 µM sense primer
>
> 1 µl 20 µM reverse primer
>
> 1 µl Taq Polymerase - Antibody complex
>
> x µl template
>
> aqua dest. to bring volume to 50 µl

The thermal cycler (*GeneAmp PCR System* / Perkin Elmar) was programmed according to the following guidelines:

- The annealing temperature depends on the sequence of the two primers. To estimate the melting temperature (T_m), the following formula was used (This simple formula works very well if the primers are between 19 bp and 28 bp in length.):

$$(A + T) \times 2 + (C + G) \times 4 = T_m$$

- The extension temperature was mainly kept at 72 °C because at this temperature Taq Polymerase has its maximum activity.
- The numbers of cycles depended mainly on the amount of template DNA in the reaction. Under normal conditions, 30 cycles are enough for a sufficient amplification. If the template sequence was expected to be rather rare, the program was run with 35 or more cycles.

To estimate the size of PCR products expected, 10 µl of the reaction was separated on an agarose gel. Described in Methods, <u>chapter 5.3.1. Agarose gel electrophoresis</u>.

7.2. Pfu Polymerase

To show evidence for a suspected polymorphism of huSCYB11 in the cell line THP-1, we amplified a part of exon 4 with Pfu polymerase. The Pfu DNA polymerase is a thermostable enzyme isolated from *Pyrococcus furiosus*. The enzyme exhibits a 5′→3′ DNA polymerase activity and a 3′→5′ exonuclease activity. This proofreading is useful for PCR reactions requiring high fidelity synthesis.

hSCYB11polys	sense	CCTTAAGAAAGGCTGGTTACCATC
hSCYB11polyr	anti-sense	AAAGTGATTGCTAGGTATACATTTGC

As a template, we took cDNA and genomic DNA, both isolated from THP-1 cells.

PCR reaction was performed as follows:

5 µl Pfu-buffer containing 20 mM MgSO$_4$

1 µl dNTP 10 mM

3 µl primer hSCYB11polys (10 mM)

3 µl primer hSCYB11polyr (10 mM)

template (cDNA or genomic DNA)

1 µl Pfu-polymerase

aqua dest. to bring volume to 50 µl

cycling parameters:

1 cycle:	2 min 95 °C
40 cycles:	30 sec 95 °C
	1 min 63 °C
	2 min 74 °C
1 cycle:	5 min 74 °C
hold at 4 °C	

After thermocycling the PCR product was purified with *Qiaquick Nucleotide Removal Kit* (Qiagen).

7.3. Genome Walking

Genome Walking is a PCR method to "walk" upstream or downstream from a known sequence into an unknown adjacent sequence part. For this approach the *Mouse Genome Walking Kit* (Clontech) was used.

The kit contains five libraries of uncloned adaptor ligated genomic DNA fragments. These libraries were constructed from genomic DNA of ICR Swiss mice by restriction with one of the five restriction enzymes (EcoRV, ScaI, DraI, PvuII or SspI) and adapters were ligated to both ends.

7.3.1. Primer design

The gene specific primers were designed according to the following rules:

- outer and nested primer should not overlap
- primer should be 25-28 nucleotides in length and have 40-60 % G/C content
- primers should not be able to anneal to the adapter primers
- not more than three Gs and Cs should occur in the last six positions of the 3´ end

gsp1.prim	outer primer	GCACCCATACCATTGTCACCTCCAGC
gsp2.prim	nested primer	CGTCGACTTTGTCGCAGCCGTTACTCG

Primers were designed from the cDNA of muCXCL11 (binding to exon 2 of genomic DNA) and extended the known sequence in 3´ direction.

mscybg3a.prim	outer primer	GTGGTCTGTCCCAGGCTTCCTTATGTTC
mscybg3i.prim	nested primer	CGAGTAACGGCTGCGACAAAGTTGAAG

Primers were designed for the genomic DNA fragment derived from the first Genome Walking experiments. Primers extended the sequence in 3´ direction and obtained the murine genomic sequence down to exon 4.

mscybg5a.prim	outer primer	GTGGAGCATTGTCAGTATCCACACTAC
mscybg5i.prim	nested primer	GATTCTCTGAACAGGCATTGAGGACTG

Primers were designed from the genomic PCR fragment derived from the first Genome Walking experiments and were used to extend the sequence in 5´ direction up to exon 1.

mscybgpa.prim	outer primer	CCAGATGATCGCAGCCAGGGCTATG
mscybgpi.prim	nested primer	GCTGTGACCTTCCTGTTCATCTCAGCA

Primers were designed from exon 1 into 5´ direction to obtain the start codon.

mscybgp2a.prim	outer primer	CATACCAGGTGACCTTCATCTATC
mscybgp2i.prim	nested primer	CTGAAACACTCTCCCCATAGCTGTAC

Primers were designed from the beginning of exon 1 into 5´ direction to obtain a part of the promoter region.

muscybg6a.prim	outer primer	GGTTACAGTGGATGCATTGTTACTGC
muscybg6i.prim	nested primer	CACGAGGCACACGAACATCTAGGAAG

Primers were designated from exon 4 into 3´ directions to obtain the end of exon 4.

The Genome Walking PCR reaction was carried out with *Advantage Genomic Polymerase Mix* (Clontech). This polymerase mix contains *Tth DNA polymerase*, a minor amount of a second DNA polymerase to provide 3´→5´ proofreading activity and *Tth Start antibody* (Clontech) to provide hot start PCR. The simultaneous use of two different DNA polymerases in a PCR reaction can permit amplification of longer fragments (= long-distance PCR).

7.3.2. Procedure for PCR-based DNA walking

The primary PCR reaction was carried out with an outer adaptor primer (AP1) provided in the kit and an outer gene-specific primer. The primary PCR reaction mixture is then used as a template for the secondary (nested) PCR reaction using the nested adaptor primer (AP2) and a nested gene-specific primer. For the gene-specific primers see Methods, chapter 7.3.1. Primer design.

The DNA fragments obtained by this procedure begin within known sequences at the 5´ ends and extend into the unknown adjacent genomic DNA. The PCR products were cloned into the *TA-cloning vector* and subsequently sequenced.

A PCR master mix combining the following reagents was prepared:

227 µl aqua dest (or 212 µl aqua dest. + 15 µl DMSO)

30 ml 10x Tth PCR reaction buffer

6 µl dNTP (10 mM each)

13.2 µl Mg(OA₂) 25 mM

6 ml AP1 primer (10 µM)

6 µl outer gene specific primer (10 µM)

6µl Advantage Genomic Polymerase Mix (Clontech)

49 µl of this PCR master mix was aliquoted into 6 Thermowell tubes on ice. 1 µl of each of the five libraries was added to the appropriate tube. In the last tube, functioning as a negative control, aqua dest was added instead of one of the libraries.

Cycling parameters:

1 cycle:	1 min 94 °C
10 cycles:	20 sec 94 °C
	4 min 68 °C
45 cycles:	20 sec 94 °C
	4 min 62 °C
1 cycle:	8 min at 62 °C
holding at 4 °C	

Touchdown PCR involves an annealing/extension temperature that is several degrees higher than the T_m of the primers. Although primer annealing is less efficient at this higher temperature it is also much more specific.

7.3.3. Secondary (nested) PCR reaction

10 µl of the primary PCR reaction products were resolved and visualized in agarose gels. When a product was obtained, 1 µl of the primary PCR reaction was taken to prepare the second amplification reaction. The PCR master mix was prepared as described for the primary PCR master mix using the nested primers AP2 and the inner gene-specific primer.

49 µl of this master mix was pipetted into each tube (stand on ice), before 1 µl of the undiluted primary PCR reaction was added. In the last tube, 1 µl of aqua dest was added (negative control). The cycle parameters were the same as for the primary reaction. 10 µl of the secondary PCR product were analysed in agarose gels, together with a DNA marker.

The PCR fragments obtained from secondary Genome Walking were cloned into the TA cloning-vector as described in Methods, chapter 6.2.2. Ligation into TA-vector.

8. Transfection

Transfection is the process of introducing nucleic acids into cells by non-viral methods. Different transfection techniques like electroporation or calcium phosphate co-precipitation have been described. For the present study a method that involved artificial liposomes (*Tfx-50* / Promega) was used. At physiological pH, these liposomes are overall positively charged. The cationic portion of the lipid molecules associates with the negatively charged nucleic acids. Furthermore the positively charged liposome allows a close association with the negatively charged cell membrane, resulting in high transfection efficiency.

Following endocytosis, the complex appears in the endosome and later in the nucleus.

8.1. Plasmid DNA for transfection

The pGL3 Luciferase reporter vector is designed for analysis of genetic regulatory elements such as promoters and enhancers. As outlined in Methods, chapter 6.2.3. Ligation into pGL3$_{basis}$ vector, the vector contains the reporter gene firefly luciferase and a part of human SCYB11 promoter. Together with the pGL3 vector, the pRL-TK (Renilla luciferase control vector) was cotransfected at a ratio of 1:5. Expression of Renilla luciferase provides an internal control value to which expression of the experimental firefly luciferase reporter gene can be normalized.

The quality of the DNA used for transfection is critical. Purified plasmid DNA should be free from LPS and chemical contaminations. For purification of the plasmid the *EndoFree*^{TM} *Plasmid Kit* (Qiagen) was used. See Methods, chapter 2.4. Endotoxin-free plasmid isolation.

8.2. Cell transfection

1×10^5 cells were transferred into each well of a *24-well plate* one day prior to transfection. The plasmid DNA (0.75 µg DNA per well) was mixed with 2.2 µl *Tfx*^{TM} *50 reagent* and brought to a final volume of 200 µl per well with serum-free medium. The DNA/ *Tfx*^{TM}*50* mixture was incubated at room temperature for 15 min. The optimal DNA / liposome ratio was determined according to the manufactures protocol.

The cell culture medium was removed and then cells were washed once with DMEM (plus glutamine but without FCS) before the transfection mixture was added. For the transfection period, the plate was returned to the incubator for another 1 hour. At the end of the transfection the cells were overlaid with 1 ml of DMEM plus 10 % FCS and glutamine (prewarmed to 37 °C) and returned to the incubator.

The transfected cells were kept for 48 hours in the incubator before cells were lysed and the luciferase activity was measured.

Stimulation

In order to test out different stimuli, the following stimuli were added 24 hours after transfection:

625 U/ml IFN-α	625 U/ml IFN-β	625 U/ml IFN-γ
500 U/ml TNF-α	1 µg/ml LPS	2.5 ng/ml IL-1β

These stimuli either were used alone or in varying combinations.

8.3. Preparation of cell lysates

Two days after transfection, the growth medium was removed from the cultured cells and they were washed in 1 ml PBS. Afterwards, 100 µl of passive lysis buffer was dispensed on the cells in each culture well.

For better lysis the plates were frozen for 30 min at -80 °C and placed on ice to let them thaw gently. The entire lysate was transferred into a 1.5 ml tube and centrifuged for 2 min at 9000 rcf. 40 µl of the supernatant were pipetted into each well of a white 96 *well chimney base* for the following assay and measurement.

8.4. Assay and measurement

To measure the enzyme activities of firefly and renilla luciferase, the *Dual-Luciferase® Reporter Assay System* (Promega) was used. The *LARII* (Luciferase assay reagent II) and *Stop&Glo* reagent were prepared as described in the manual.

The firefly luciferase reporter is measured first by adding *LARII* to generate a "glow-type" luminescent signal. After quantifying the firefly luminescence, this reaction is quenched and the Renilla luciferase reaction is initiated by simultaneously adding *Stop&Glo reagent* to the same probe. The Stop&Glo reagent also produces a "glow-type" signal from Renilla luciferase.

The assay was performed in white 96 *well chimney bases*. The *Liquid Scintillation & Luminescence Counter* was equipped with two reagent injectors for a sequential injection of the *LARII* and *Stop&Glo reagents*. The activity of firefly luciferase was determined by injecting 40 µl *LARII*. After a 2 sec premeasurement delay, a 5 sec measurement period followed. Subsequently, 40 µl *Stop&Glo reagent* was injected. Again, after 2 sec of premeasurement, a 5 sec measurement period followed.

The relative firefly luciferase activity for each assay was calculated as the percentage of that of renilla luciferase activity.

III. Results

1. Characterization of human CXCL11

1.1. Isolation of CXCL11 cDNA

A cDNA library, prepared from poly-A$^+$ RNA isolated from THP-1 myelomonocytoma cells, treated for 7 hours with 250 U/ml IFN-γ, was screened for GTP cyclohydrolase I.

GTP cyclohydrolase I is a cytokine-inducible enzyme involved in biosynthesis of the cofactor tetrahydrobiopterin (Werner ER et al. 1998). Various clones were isolated and analysed from the library. One clone was found to contain a second reading frame encoding a CXC chemokine. Sequence analysis (Wisconsin Sequence Analysis Package of the Genetics Computer Group [GCG], Madison, WI) showed that this second reading frame was linked to the GTP cyclohydrolase I cDNA via the EcoRI linker used for cloning into the Lambda Zap II vector (Stratagene). This linker was used for the construction of the library and obviously the second reading frame remained linked to the GTP cyclohydrolase I most likely due to insufficient EcoRI digestion.

The cDNA of the chemokine (later termed SCYB11 / CXCL11) had not been identified at these days. Both genes, GTP cyclohydrolase I and CXCL11 have in common that they are expressed in monocytes / macrophages upon stimulation with IFN-γ.

A 1520 bp fragment containing the CXCL11 cDNA and flanking vector sequences was isolated by SmaI restriction digestion and subcloned into the

Bluescript II SK⁻ vector. The sequence was confirmed by cycle sequencing. A 1445 bp sequence was submitted to GenBank (Accession No. U66096).

1.2. Analysis of human CXCL11 cDNA

1.2.1. Characteristic sites found in human CXCL11 cDNA

Start codon and Kozak sequence

The sequence around the ATG codon is important for the correct initiation of translation by eukaryotic ribosomes. The start codon of human CXCL11 cDNA is surrounded by the nucleotide sequence AAC**ATG**AG (shown in *Figure 6*). According to the rule for optimal sequence initiation (A -3/G +4) the purine in position -3 would allow an initiation of translation with high probability (Kozak M 1986).

Polyadenylation Sites

The CXCL11 cDNA clone contains a potential polyadenylation site AATAAA 27 nucleotides before the 3´end (see *Figure 6*). In general, AAUAAA is by far the most predominant element for direct cleavage and polyadenylation of preRNA, although minor specific nucleotide substitutions are found (Birnstiel ML et al. 1985).

A comparison of CXCL11 cDNA isolated from other cell types (e.g. astrocytoma cell line (Rani MSR et al. 1996, Cole KE et al. 1998) and PBMC (Jacobs KA et al. 1997)) showed the usage of different polyadenylation sites. These polyadenylation signals with different strength are in tandem orientation in the 3´ UTR region.

AREs for rapid mRNA degradation

Adenylate/uridylate-rich elements (AREs) are found in the 3´ untranslated region (UTR) of many mRNAs that code for cytokines, proto-oncogenes and nuclear transcription factors. Human CXCL11 cDNA contains in the 3´ UTR-region several T-rich domains, T stretches, and the pentanucleotide ATTTA, which may indicate the presence of AREs. These motifs are responsible for rapid and selective mRNA degradation and thus play a role in the regulation of gene expression in the immune response and differentiation (Chen CYA and Shyu AB 1995).

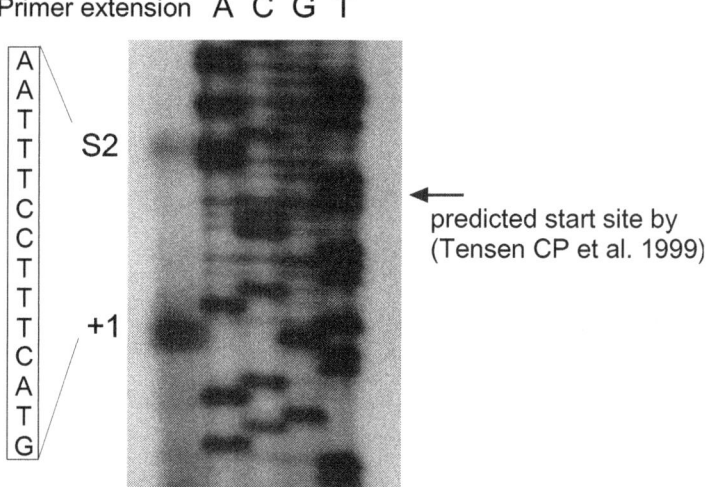

Figure 4: Primer extension

Identification of transcription start sites in CXCL11 by primer extension analysis. Reference lanes labelled A, C, G, T depict the sequence obtained with the same primer as in the primer extension sample. The two start sites are indicated as +1 (the main transcription start site) and S2. The start site predicted by Tensen CP et a. (1999b) is indicated by an arrow.

1.2.2. Start of the cDNA (primer extension)

The 5′ end of huCXCL11 cDNA was mapped by primer extension analysis. A reverse primer migtrans.prim (listed in Methods, <u>chapter 6.6. Primer extension</u>) binding in exon 1 and total RNA isolated from THP-1 cells stimulated with 1250 U/ml IFN-γ and 1 µg LPS was used. As is shown in *Figure 4*, two major labelled products were obtained, suggesting that transcription of CXCL11 is initiated from at least two sites, at nucleotide +1 and -12. The most frequent site appears to be at nucleotide +1 (the double band in *Figure 4*). The use of various transcription start sites is also known from other genes (Ogg SL et al. 1996).

A predicted transcription start site was described by (Tensen CP et al. 1999b) which is between the two determined sites at -9. This start site was deduced according to the rule that the start of transcription is roughly 25 bp behind the TATA-box (Stryer L 1996).

1.2.3. Analysis of the pre-mRNA

On Northern blots, the huCXCL11 mRNA gave a major signal at 1.7 kb and two weaker signals at 4.6 kb and 2.8 kb, as was estimated by comparison with the migrated distance of 18 S and 28 S ribosomal RNA bands (1.9 kb and 4.8 kb, respectively) (Laich A et al. 1999). The 4.6 kb signal was clearly visible upon IFN-γ treatment but also was seen with high doses of other IFNs after prolonged exposure. The expression pattern of CXCL11 on Northern blots is shown in *Figure 1* in Introduction, chapter 2.4. Expression of CXCL11.

We confirmed the 4.6 kb and 2.8 kb bands as unspliced and partial spliced pre-mRNAs, by Northern blot analysis, using a part of intron1 (huSCYBINT1) as a probe. The probe is listed in Methods, chapter 5.5.1. List of probes. Labelling with this probe gave a strong signal for the 4.6 kb unspliced pre-mRNA band. Also the 2.8 kb band was weakly visible, suggesting that this band is partially spliced pre-mRNA. The main band (1.7 kb), which could not be labelled with this intron 1 probe, is the correctly spliced mRNA of CXCL11 (data not shown).

1.2.4. Polymorphism

Partial and full-length sequences of human CXCL11 were isolated by various investigators from different cell types: human astrocytoma cells (Rani MSR et al. 1996,

Cole KE et al 1998), human primary fetal PBMC (Jacobs KA et al. 1997), and THP-1 cells (Laich A et al. 1999).

Comparing these cDNAs, we observed a sequence variation in the THP-1 cDNA within the 3´ UTR (untranslated regions) of exon 4 and exon 1. Therefore we looked for a polymorphism by direct sequencing of the amplified exon 4 from genomic and cDNA isolated from THP-1 cells with Pfu-polymerase. The PCR product was directly sequenced and analysed with GCG, confirming the polymorphism.

In exon 4, we obtained 3 transitions from G to A and two transitions from A to G. In this case, a purine was exchanged by the other purine. Furthermore, we found 4 transitions from T to C and one from C to T (change from one pyrimidine to the other). A single transversion from C to A (change from a purine to a pyrimidine) was also found. In exon 1, a single transition was found exchanging an A to G. All nucleotide exchanges are graphically represented in *Figure 5*. They are all predicted to be silent, since none of them occurs within the coding region.

A polymorphism in the 3´-noncoding region is also reported for the mouse CXCL10 mRNA isolated from mice of the C57BL/6 strain in comparison to mRNA isolated from BALB/c and MRL mice (Hallensleben W et al. 2000).

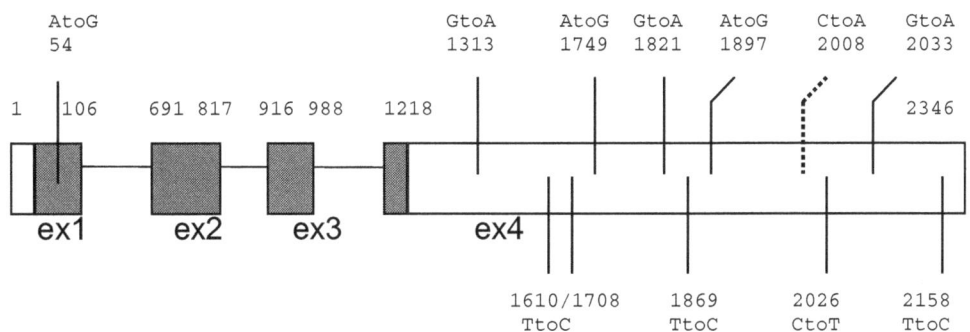

Figure 5: Polymorphism of CXCL11 obtained in THP-1 cells

The general structure of the gene is shown as boxes (exons) and the interrupted line denoting introns. The numbers indicate the range of the exons. The lines show the relative position of point mutations obtained in THP-1 myelomonocytoma cells. The transitions are shown as solid lines, the single transversion is shown as a hatched line.

1.3. Isolation of the genomic SCYB11 sequence

SCYB11 specific PCR primers (migbse1.prim and migbse2.prim listed in Methods, chapter 7.1.2. List of primers) were used to amplify a 268 bp fragment from THP-1 cells genomic DNA. The fragment contained a part of exon 2, intron 3 and a part of exon 3. (GenBank Accession No. AF053972)

Under the same PCR conditions, a PAC library was screened (Genome Systems, St. Louis, Missouri). Two positive clones were isolated PAC: 17352 and PAC 17353. The DNA of the PAC 17352 was purified as described in Methods, chapter 2.3. PAC and BAC isolation, and restriction digested with EcoRI, PstI, and HincII. Positive fragments were identified after Southern blotting and hybridized with the probe mg, which is listed in Methods, chapter 5.5.1. List of probes.

The positive EcoRI (~1.7 kb) fragment contains of 311 bp of the promoter region and spans the sequence of exon 1 to exon 4. The fragment terminates 81 bp behind the STOP codon. The PstI fragment (~3.5 kb) starts within exon 4, namely 340 bp behind the STOP codon and extends 2800 bp into the region behind the gene. The missing sequence fragment of exon 4 was amplified by PCR with the primer pair migse1.prim and huscyb11gen2.prim (listed in Methods, chapter 7.1.2. List of primers). Sequence data were analysed using GCG. The complete genomic sequence was submitted to GenBank (Accession No. AF077867).

To analyse the promoter region, PAC 17352 was restriction digested with HincII. The positive fragment (~3,8 kb) was subcloned into Blueskript SK⁻. The fragment spans 3433 bp of the promoter region and terminates at + 438 bp in intron 1.

In summary, 8799 bp were subcloned from PAC 17352, custom sequenced and analysed with GCG. The complete sequence is listed in *Figure 6*.

```
-3433  AACTCATCTTTTATTAAGTGGTTGTGTTTGTGTTAATGCTGAAAAACAGCTGAAAACAAGCTAGATGTGGTATGCCAATT
-3353  CAGGAAAGGACACTGATAATAATAATAGCAGTTAATACATTTTGAGTGCTACATATTTTTCTAAATGATTAATATGCATT
                NF-ATc        GATA-1                                       NF-IL6
-3273  ACCTCTTTTAATACCTAGTTTATAACAGCCCTATGAAAAAGGGGTCTGAGACCAGCCTGGCCAACATGGTGAAACCCCAT
-3193  CTCTACTAAAAATACAAAAATTGGCTGGGCGTGGTAACACATGCCTGTCATCCCAGCTACTTGGGAGGCTGAGGCAAGAC
-3113  AATCGCTTGAACCCAGGAGGCGGAGGTTGCAGTAAGCCGAGATCATGCCACTGCACTCCAGCCTGGGTGGCACAGAGAGA
-3033  CTCCATCTCAAAAAAAAAAAAAAAAGTACTATTATTATCCCCAGTCTATAGATGAGAAAATAGCCTCAAAAAGTTGCGGTA
                                         GATA-1
-2953  ACTTGTTCATAAATAACTGAATGTGGGCTGGGCACAGTGGCTCACGCCTGTAATCCCAGCACTTTGGGAGGCCAAGGCGG
-2873  CAGGATCACCTGAGGTTAGGAGTTCAAGACCAGCTTGGCCAACATGGCTAAACACCATCTCTACTAAAAACTATAAAAATT
-2793  AGCCAGGCATGGAGGCACGCACCTGTAATCCCAGCTACTTGGGAGGCTGAGGCAGGCGAATCACTTGAATCCACGAGGCA
-2713  GAGGCTGTGGTGAGTCGAGATCACACCACTGCACTCCAGCCTGGGGCTACAGAGCAAGAACCCATCTCAAAGATAAATAA
                                                                          GATA-1
-2633  ATAAATAAATAAATAAATAATCAAGGGTGGATTTGAACACAAGCTGACTCTAGAGCCTTCCCTATTAACAACTATGCTCT

                            ⟹
-2553  ACTGTGTTTCTAATGCTGAGAAAATGAAAAGCAACATTAAAAAATAATAACAGATAAGGATTTATGAGCTCCAAGAACAC
                                                        GATA-1
-2473  ATTCCTTTTACTTTACCCATATTCCTGAGGGAAAATTAGTCTTTCTTTACATATGTTAAATGAATTAATGGAAAAGAAGG
-2393  AAAGAATATTCCAGCTACTTGGAAATTAATTAAAATACAGTAGCCCCCTCACCTTATCCTTGGGGGATATGTTCCAAGAC
                                                         GATA-1
-2313  CCCCAATGAGTGCCTGAAACTGCAGATAGTACTGAGCCCTGTATATATTGTATTTTTTCCTGTACATATATACCTATAAA
                             GATA-1
-2233  AAAGTTTGATTTATAAATTAGCCACAGTAAGAGCATCAACATTAATATATAGAATAATTACAACAATATTCTGTAATAAA
-2153  ACTTAAGTGACTGTGTAGTCTCTCTCTCTTCAAATATCTTATTGTACTATACTCACTCTTCTAGTGATGCTGTGAAATGA
              AP-1
-2073  TAAAATGTCTATGTGATGGGATGAAGTGATGGAGCAAGATGATGTGAGATTTCATCATGCTACTCAGAAAAGTGCTTAAA
                                                       NF-IL6
-1993  ACTTATGAATTATTTCTAGAATTTCTCATTTAATGGGGGACTACTGTAAAGACTTTCAAAGGTTTTAAAGACTAGTCATG
-1913  GTTGTTAAAGAATTTAAATGCAGGATTATATCTAAATAAATATACAATTTCAAGATAAAATGCAAATGATAATTCTCAAA
                                                   GATA-1
-1833  AAAAGAAGTTGAATAAGATAAAATAATAATCTAAAAGTAATAAACTGGCTATAAATTCCCCGATTATACCAACTTTTATT
              GATA-1
-1753  GGTAAAACTAGGAAATAGGAGAAAATTCTTGAAAGAAAGTTACAGTGATTTTCTCATGTTACAAAGACAGGAGCTAAAAA
```

```
-1673   AATATCATTGATGGTTGATGTAAATAATTAGAAAAATTCAGGTAAAAATCTTTTTAAAGAATTTTAAGAATTAATATCAA
-1593   AATGTAAAACAATGTATTCCTTTCAAATTACTTAAGGAAGGCCAAGCACCGTGGCTCATCCCAGTAATCCTAGCACTTTG
                               NF-IL6                                    ⟹
-1513   GGAGACCAAGGCAGGAGGATTGCTTGAGGCCTGGAGTTCATGGCTGCAGTGAGCTACGATTGTGCCACTCGACTCCAGAA
-1433   TGGTGACAGAGTGAGACCCATCTCATTAAAAAAAACAAAAATGGCTTCAAAAAGTTAAATAAAATATATTTAAAGTTAGA
          AP-1
-1353   AAGAAATCAAAGAAAAACATAAAGAATCAGCAAGGAAGCATTTTAAAAATTACAGATTACCAGTTATACAGTAAATATATT
-1273   TTATTACGCTTACCCATTAGAAAGCTCCTTTGATATGATTTTCTTAAACATCTACAAGTGACACACTTAAAACAAAGATT
                                  GATA-1              AP-1
-1193   TAGGAAGCTTAAGAGGAAAGATAAAGACAAAAAAATAGGAATTACATCAAAGTAGAATCTCAGAGGTAAAACTATCACAT
          NF-IL6        GATA-1                                           GATA-1
-1113   GAGCAAAGACGATCACTTTTTTTTATGAACCCTAATACAACTCATACAACTTCATGTACTAAGTAACAGTGCTAAAATAT
-1033   ATATAAAGTAGCTTTCCACCATGGCCACCATTGGAGGGCAGCAGCCATGACACTGCACTACCCTATAGCTGTGGGCCTCA
-953    ACAAGGGCCACAAGGTGACCAAGAATGTGAGCAAGCCCAGGCACAGCCACTGTGGGCGCCTGACCAAACTCACTAAATTT
                        AP-1
-873    GTGTGGGACATGATCCCAGAGGTGTGTGGCTTCACCCCTAACGAGTGGCGTGGCATGGAGTTACTGAAGGTCTCCAAGGT
-793    CAAACAGGCCCTCAAATTCATCAAGAAAAGGGTAGGGACAAACATCTGCGCCAAGAGAAGGCAGGAGGAGCTGAGCAACG
-713    TCCTGGCTGCCATGAGGAAAGCAGCTGCCAAGAAGGACTGAGCCCCCTGCCATCTGCCTATAATGAAAGCTTTGCAGAAT
                                                                       NF-IL6
-633    AAAATAAATATAAAATAAAGTAATAAAATTAAATTTAAAAATAAAATAAAGCAAAACAAAATAAAATATATAAAGTAAAA
                                                                   OCT-1
-553    ATTGTTGAAAATGCAAAACAATATGGACATAAATACAGAAACACAGGGAAACTTCTTTAGGCACTCATTTACAGGTAAAA
          NF-IL6
-473    ATATGAAATTGAATAAAGGTCATCTGGTGTCAAATAATATAGGCCTTATCTATTATAAGAGTTTGGACTGAAAAGCAAAA
                                             GATA-1        ⟹              IRF-1/IFR-2
-393    GTGAGATAATAAAAAAAAGCTTTTCAGAATATTATTTTGTATAGATATGTGAAGGATGAAAGGTGGGTGAAAGGACCAAA
                               NF-IL6             GATA-1
-313    AACAGAAACACAGTCTTCCTGAATGAATGACAATCAGAATTCCGCTGCCCAAAGTAGTCCGACAATTAAATGGATTTCTA
          IRF-1   /OCT1 ⟹    AP-1
-233    GGAAAAGCTACCTTAAGAAGGCTGGTTACCATCTGGGTTTTCACAGTGCTTTCACATTCTTATCACTTTCAACACTACTG
          GAS                                        NF-IL6      GATA-1
-153    CAAATAGGAAGGGACAGTAACATTTAGAAGAGAACAAAACAGAAACTCTTGGAAGCAGGAAAGGTGCATGACTCAAAGAG
                               ISRE/IRF-1                               AP-1
-73     GGAAATTCCTGTGCCATAAAAGGATTGCTGGTGTATAAAATGCTCTATATATGCCAATTATCAATTTCCTTTCATGTTCA
          NF-κB                        TATA-box  TATA-box  CAAT  S2        +1
7       GCATTTCTACTCCTTCCAAGAAGAGCAGCAAAGCTGAAGTAGCAGCAACAGCACCAGCAGCAACAGCAAAAAACAAACAT
                                                                                    M
87      GAGTGTGAAGGGCATGGCTATAGCCTTGGCTGTGATATTGTGTGCTACAGTTGTTCAAGGTATGCAGTAATTTTTATTTC
         S   V   K   G   M   A   I   A   L   A   V   I   L   C   A   T   V   V   Q
```

167   TCAACCTATAAGTTCCTTTTCTAATGTTTCAAATGTCTTTTCTTCCACTTTTATCCTAAAAGACATGATAAAGTTTTATT

247   TAATCTCACAGATTAGAAGTTACTACAGCTTTAGCACAGAAATGGTGGACATGTTTAAGATACTAGAGATGATTATTGAA

327   ACTAGAAATTATGAACTTCATGGAATTTTTGATTTGGCTAGAATATCTGGCAAAAGCCTTTAGCAACAGTTTTAAATGTC

407   TGTTAAGAAGATTTTATATAGCGATCATGTTAACAAGCTTCCTGGGAAAATATTTGAGGATAAAATCAAGGGGGCAAAAC

487   AAGCTTCACCTCCAATAAACTTCCTTCATGCTTCCCATTTGTTAGCGATTTGCTTACTAATTTAATGAGAAAATAATCAA

567   CATCTTACTTAACTTTTCCCAGTAACAGATGTGTTAAGTGCTATTTGACAAATTACTATCTTTACCCTTAATGAAAATTC

647   TGCTCACGTTCACCACCAGCTATAAACCACAGCCATCTGTTGCAATCAGACGCATTACTAACTAATGCTATGATCTATTC

727   TAG**GCTTCCCCATGTTCAAAAGAGGACGCTGTCTTTGCATAGGCCCTGGGGTAAAAGCAGTGAAAGTGGCAGATATTGAG**
        G P M F K R G R C L C I G P G V K A V K V A D I E

807   **AAAGCCTCCATAATGTACCCAAGTAACAACTGTGACAAAATAGAAGTGAT**GTAAGTAATGAACTTGCTGAAGATGACAAT
      K A S I M Y P S N N C D K I E V I

887   GGTGCAGGCTTTTTTGTTTATGTATTTGCATCTAAACTTTAAGACTCTTTTGTATGTTCTTTTAACAG**TATTACCCTGAA**
                                                                  I T L K

967   **AGAAAATAAAGGACAACGATGCCTAAATCCCAAATCGAAGCAAGCAAGGCTTATAATCAAA**GTAAGTTACCAGATTACTC
      E N K G Q R C L N P K S K Q A R L I I K

1047   CCATGTTATAATCTGTTTTATCCAAGACAGATCTTTTGAAAAAGAAAATAATGTGGACAACTACAGAAAGATTCTGCTAT

1127   GATCCTGTGTGAAATATTCTGTTAAGGGGTCCTTGGTTGTAACAGCTTCCCCTTCTTACTACATGTTTTTAGATGTCCTG

1207   GGGGAAACAAGAACAGCCCAAGTAAATAAAACTCTTGTTTTCTTATTCCAG**AAAGTTGAAAGAAAGAATTTTTAAAAATA**
                                                              K V E R K N F *

1287   **TCAAAACATATGAAGTCCTGGAAAAGGGCATCTGAAAAACCTAGAACAAGTTTAACTGTGACTACTGAAATGACAAGAAT**

1367   **TCTACAGTAGGAAACTGAGACTTTTCTATGGTTTTGTGACTTTCAACTTTTGTACAGTTATGTGAAGGATGAAAGGTGGG**
1447   **TGAAAGGACCAAAAACAGAAATACAGTCTTCCTGAATGAATGACAATCAGAATTCCACTGCCCAAAGGAGTCCAACAATT**
1527   **AAATGGATTTCTAGGAAAAGCTACCTTAAGAAAGGCTGGTTACCATCGGAGTTTACAAAGTGCTTTCACGTTCTTACTTG**
1607   **TTGTATTATACATTCATGCATTTCTAGGCTAGAGAACCTTCTAGATTTGATGCTTACAACTATTCTGTTGTGACTATGAG**
1687   **AACATTTCTGTCTCTAGAAGTTATCTGTCTGTATTGATCTTTATGCTATATTACTATCTGTGGTTACAGTGGAGACATTG**
1767   **ACATTATTACTGGAGTCAAGCCCTTATAAGTCAAAAGCACCTATGTGTCGTAAAGCATTCCTCAAACATTTTTTCATGCA**
1847   **AATACACACTTCTTTCCCCAAATATCATGTAGCACATCAATATGTAGGGAAACATTCTTATGCATCATTTGGTTTGTTTT**
1927   **ATAACCAATTCATTAAATGTAATTCATAAAATGTACTATGAAAAAAAATTATACGCTATGGGATACTGGCAACAGTGCACA**

```
2007  TATTTCATAACCAAATTAGCAGCACCGGTCTTAATTTGATGTTTTTCAACTTTTATTCATTGAGATGTTTTGAAGCAATT
2087  AGGATATGTGTGTTTACTGTACTTTTTGTTTTGATCCGTTTGTATAAATGATAGCAATATCTTGGACACATTTGAAATAC
2167  AAAATGTTTTTGTCTACCAAAGAAAAATGTTGAAAAATAAGCAAATGTATACCTAGCAATCACTTTTACTTTTTGTAATT
2247  CTGTCTCTTAGAAAAATACATAATCTAATCAATTTCTTTGTTCATGCCTATATACTGTAAAATTTAGGTATACTCAAGAC
2327  TAGTTTAAAGAATCAAAGTCATTTTTTTCTCTAATAAACTACCACAACCTTTCTTTTTTAAAAAAAGATCTATATACTTT
                                         poly A site
2407  CCAGGACATTTGAGATGCCTTTAACAATTTTGCCTTATATTTCAGAAACATACACCTATCCGTCATCATGAAAAACTGTT
2487  TAGAAATATATTTTAATGGGTAGGTGGGAAAGACAGTTGTTTCTTTTGTCGGCCTTGGGGGGTCTTGATAGTCCAAACCC
2567  CCTTCTTACTTGGAGAAAATCCCTTATGTGAGTGTTGGTGGGAGGCCAAAAGAGAGAAGCCAAAGACAGGAGATCCTCTC
2647  CTGTAGCCACAACAAGGACTCAGCCATGCTGTTTCTACCCTAGACTTTGAACTCCAGCTGGCATCACAAAGATACTATTA
2727  GTAAGAAAATTATTTCAAGCCTGGCAGCAGCAGGAGAAACAATGAAAGTCTTACAGTAGTGTCTTCCCAATGTGTGTTCC
2807  TGTAGCATGACTCCGGCTAGTCCTTCCTATCACCTAGTTCCCTTAGGTCTTTGTCCATTTTCCAAGACTTATTCTCCATT
2887  GTCCTGTGGATTCTTCAACCTCCAACTAAATTCTTTTTCTCCTTAAGTAGCCAGAGTTGGTTTCTCTGCATGTAACCAA
2967  AAGCCTTGACTGATAGCAGTACTCTCTATATAGGCACCCATACATTTGAAAAATAAAAATATTTATTATAGGATTATAAT
3047  CAGATATATCTGTATTGCATTATTATATAGGTTATAGATACAATATAGATTTATAATAAATTGTTATATAAATCTATATA
3127  AATATCTATATAGAGATGGGACTTCCATATAAATTCCCTGGATAGTTTTAAGACCTGAATCTGGCTGGGTGCGATGGCTC
3207  ACATCTGTAATCCCAGCACTTTGGGAGGCCGAAGCGGGCGGATCACCTGAGGTCAGGAGTTCAAGACCAGCATGGCTAAC
3287  ATGGTGAAACCCCATTTCTACTTAAAATGCAAAAAATTAGCCGAGTGTGCTGGCATGTGCCTGTAATCCCAGCTACTCAG
3367  GAAGCTGAGGCAGGAGAATCGCTTGAACCCGGGAGGCAGAGGTTGCAGTGAGCTGAGATCATGCCATTGCATTCCAGCTT
3447  GGGCAACAAGAGTGAAACTCCACCTCAAAAAAAAAAAAAAAAAAGACTTGAATCTAATCTTTGACTACTTACAGTGATTTT
3527  TTTTTTAAGTCTCTTTAAAAATAAAAATTCACATAGTCAGCTGGGCATGGTGGCTCACACCTATAATCTGAGCACTTTGG
3607  GAGACCGACATAGGTGAATGGCTTAAGCCCAGGAGTTCAAGACTAGCTTGGGCAACATAGCGAAAATTCATCTCTATAAA
3687  AAAATATGAAAATTAGCTGGGTATGGTGGCACATGCCTGTGACCTCAGCTACTTGGGAAGCTGAGGTGGATGGATCACTTG
3767  GGTCTGGGAGGTTGAGGCTGCAGTCAGCTGTGATCACACCACTGCACTCCAGCCTGGGCAAAAGCCTGCCTCAAAAAAAA
3847  AAAAAAATTCACAGAGTTAAGGCTGCATGATAAATTGGTATTTGTAAGAAGTATATTAAATATTATAGGCCAGTACATTA
3927  TTATTGAGAAGAAAACATACACCTAAAGTTCTTCATAGCAAAATAAATATATGAAATATTAATAATTAACATATTTGAGC
4007  CAAGATCCTCCCCACCTTGGTACCTTTGCACATACTATTCTCTCTGCCCATTTCTTCACTAAGCTAATGCCTACTAATTG
4087  CTTAGGTCTCAGCTTAAATGACTTTTTCTCCAAGAAGCCTTTGAAACCACCACTTCAGCTTCAACTAGATTAGGTGTCCT
4167  ATTTATTTATTTCCATAACACTCTCTATTTTTCCATCATACTACTTACTGCAATTGTAATTAATGAATTATTCCTGTGCC
4247  TAATATCTGCTCTCTCATAAGTGTAAAAGAAAGCTGCTGTAGCCCAGGCCAACAGTACAGTTTCTGGTGCATATCAGACC
4327  CTATTGAATGGCAATATAAGCTAAGGGAAAAGGAATTTACAGCAGAGGAATGACACAAGGGAATGTACAGTAGTAGGAAG
4407  TATAAAGTGATTTTTAGGAATCATAATTAGATTCGTTTGGTTGGAAGGATGAAGGACATGAAACTGTAAATAACCTTGAA
4487  TTTTACTCTGTACAAAATGGGGATTCAATAAATGTTTGTGAAGAAGAGAGTGACCCTATCAAAGTCATTGGAAAATATTC
4567  TGGGAATTGCATGAATGGTTGATTGAAAGTGGGAAAGAGTGGAGGAGGAAAATCAGTTGGGATTTGCTGCAATAGCTGCA
4647  ATATCTCAGGTCTGTATTTCCAAAACTTCAAGGCATTCTCATATCATCTTTACAATTTTTTTTAACATTTCTCTGTTTGA
4727  TCTTCATTATATTTTTAGAAACTCTGTATACCACTTTATTTTACGTACATTTACATGAAAAGTAAACTTTCACTACTGTA
4807  CATGTAAAATCGGTAATACATGCCATGGAAATAAAATGTAATGATAAAACAAAATACAACGCAAAAATACTAATATTCCC
4887  CCTGATTTAATTAATCAGAGGGATTGAAGTTAAGAAGAGAATAATTCACCGATACTACATGTTATTATCAATGTACATGG
4967  TAGTGTCCCACACTTTGGGAAACACTGGTGTGAAAAGTAATGGGGCTGGCTCTGCAATAAGTTAAACATAATTATAGTAA
```

```
5047   TTATATATTACTATATAATCCAGCAATTCCATTCCTAGGTATATACCCAAAAGAACTGAAACAGCTCTTTAAACAAAAAC
5127   TGGTACACAAATGTTCATAGCAGCATTATACACAACAGCCAGAAAGCAGAAACAACCCAAATATCCATCAACAAGTGAAT
5207   GGATAAAATGTGGTATACACACACAATAGATTATTCGGCCATAAAAAGGAATGAAGTACTGATACATGCTACAACATGGA
5287   TGAACCTTGAAAATATGCTAAGTAAAAAAAGCCAGACACAAGGGACCACATATTGTATGATTCCATTTTATAGGAAATA
```

Figure 6: Genomic sequence of human SCYB11

Numbers on the left are relative to the main transcription initiation site (+1). The other transcription start site is indicated as S2. Underlined sequences correspond to known transcription factor binding sites. The cDNA is presented in bold letters with the poly A$^+$ site underlined. The deduced amino acid sequence is written below the cDNA.

1.4. Analysis of the promoter region

1.4.1. Computer assisted analysis of transcription factor binding sites

The genomic sequence 5´of the human CXCL11 gene was analysed up to -3433 bp with MatInspector (http://genomatrix.gsf.de), a program to detect transcription factor binding sites. The program was run with a selected subset of matrices taken from transcription factor database (TRANSFAC) (http://transfac.gbf.de.TRANSFAC). The used matrices are listed in Appendix, 1. List of regulatory elements found in the promoter region.

The computer-assisted inspection of the 5´ region revealed several consensus sequence motifs known to be involved in transcriptional regulation. The SCYB11 promoter contains one CAAT and two TATA boxes. There are several different IFN-responsive elements in a region 400 bp next to the transcription start site: an ISRE (IFN-stimulated response element) binding site is found at position -106 and a GAS site (γ-activated sequence) at position -226 bp. These sites were also identified by (Rani SMR et al. 1999, Tensen CP et al. 1999b). ISRE functions through binding the ISGF3 complex consisting of STAT1α and/or β, STAT2 and p48, while GAS elements bind the STAT1α homodimer (reviewed by Sen GC and Lengyel P 1992).

We further could detect two IRF recognition sequences at position -304 bp and at position -393 bp. The factors IRF-1 and IRF-2 are described to bind to identical cis-elements within type I IFN and IFN-inducible genes. IRF-1 functions as a transcriptional activator, while IFR-2 represses the IRF-1 function. (Takanka N et al. 1993).

A single NF-κB site was detected at position -65. A synergistic effect of the NF-κB site and the IFN responsive sites could be supposed since this was shown for murine *Scyb10* and *Scyb9* (Ohmori Y and Hamilton TA 1993, Ohmori Y et al. 1997). The characteristic γ-RE motif found in the promoter region of mouse *Scyb9* (Wong P et al. 1994) is not present in human SCYB11. Several NF-IL 6 sites (an activator induced by LPS or inflammatory proteins) were also found. NF-IL6 is also repetitively found in the promoter of murine SCYB10 (Ohmori Y and Hamilton TA 1993).

In general, the human SCYB11 promoter shows a similar picture as human and murine SCYB10 with positive promoter elements (especially IFN-γ) next to the transcription start site and negative regulatory elements in distal regions (Majumder S et al. 1998, Ohmori Y and Hamilton TA 1993).

1.4.2. Functional promoter analysis

A functional promoter analysis was carried out with a series of 5´deletion fragments which were cloned into pGL3$_{basis}$ *Luciferase Reporter vector* (Promega). The five promoter fragments used comprise base -3433 to +35, -2601 to +35, -1520 to +35, -409 to +35 and -301 to +35 of the genomic DNA shown in *Figure 6*. All pGL3 constructs were cotransfected with pRL-TK *Renilla luciferase plasmid* using *Tfx-50* (Promega) into the HepG2 cells. 24 hours after transfection, the cells were stimulated with IFN-α (625 U/ml), IFN-β (625 U/ml), IFN-γ (625 U/ml), LPS (1 µg/ml), a combination of IFN-γ and LPS, IL-1β (2.5 µg/ml), TNF-α (500 U/ml), a combination of TNF-α and LPS, or a combination of IL-1β and TNF-α. After further 24 hours, cells were lysed and relative firefly luciferase activity and renilla luciferase activity were analysed with the Dual-luciferase Reporter System (Promega). The firefly activity for three parallel assays were normalized to renilla luciferase measured in the same samples. From three parallel assays, the mean was calculated. The values presented in *Figure 7* are the average from at least two independent experiments (standard deviation is shown as whiskers).

Functional promoter analysis showed that the most important regulatory elements are close to the transcription start site. The highest induction of luciferase activity was observed in response to IFN-γ. IFN-β as a single stimulus was also a good inducer while IFN-α showed only weak effects. LPS alone or in combination with IFN-γ or TNF-α had no significant stimulatory effects (data not shown).

The promoter fragment of 440 bp showed a reduced induction by IFN-γ while the combination of IL-1β and TNF-α was a very good inducer. The promoter fragments of 1500 bp and 2600 bp showed no significant induction of luciferase activity by any of the tested stimuli, which suggested that distal elements between -2660 bp and -1500 bp negatively regulate the response to IFN-γ. Interestingly, the -3400 bp fragment showed a significant response upon stimulation with IFN-γ. Elements in this distant region could possibly compensate the effect of the reduced promoter fragments.

In general a good induction of luciferase activity was obtained upon stimulation with IFNs and IL-1 plus TNF-α, while LPS and IL-1β alone showed no significant luciferase activity. Furthermore, costimulation with IFN-γ and LPS showed no synergistic effects.

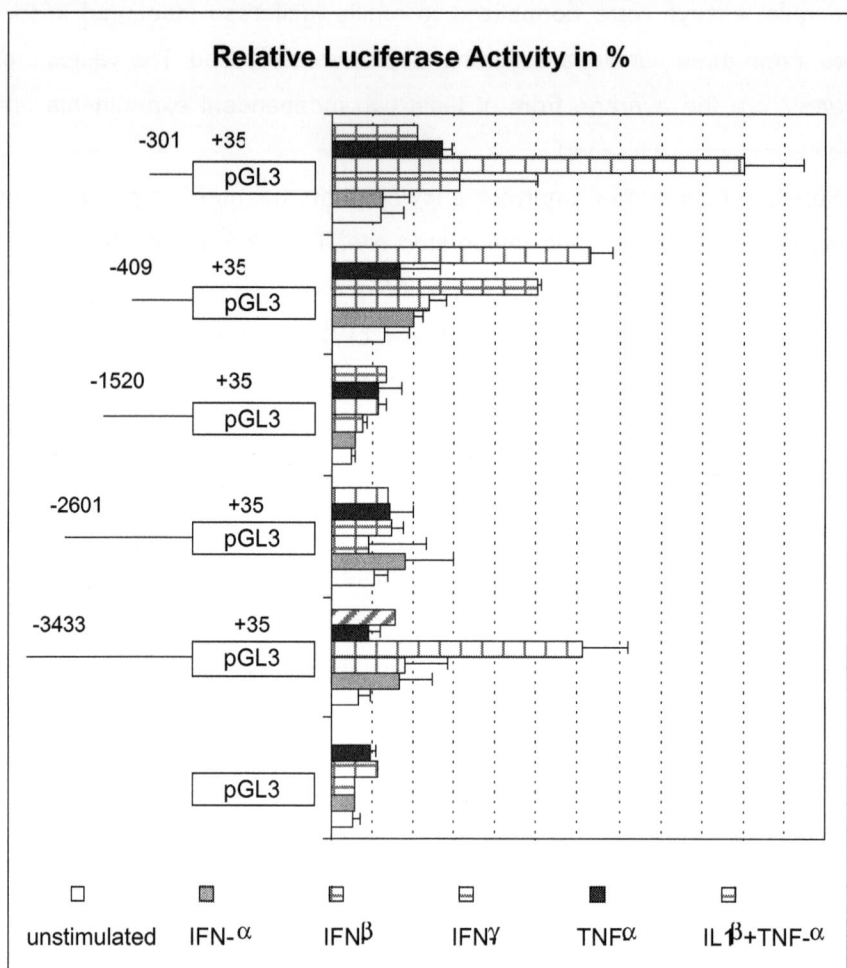

Figure 7: Functional promoter analyse

Serial 5´deletion fragments between -3433 bp and +35 bp of the human SCYB11 genomic sequence were cloned into a pGL3$_{basis}$ vector. On the left side is a schematic representation of pGL3$_{basis}$ / huSCYB11 constructs and on the right side are normalized luciferase activities determined by the *dual-luciferase reporter assay*. The relative luciferase activity is presented as percentage of activity obtained from cells transfected with the pGL3 -301 bp to +35 bp plasmid stimulated with IFN-γ. Values indicate the induction of firefly luciferase activity stimulated with IFN-α, IFN-β, IFN-γ, TNF-α, a combination of IL-1β and TNF-α versus untreated but transfected Hep-G2 cells. The values presented are the mean of at least two independent experiments and whiskers indicate the standard deviation.

1.5. Comparison of the genomic structure of SCYB11, SCYB9 and SCYB10

Comparing the intron/exon structure of SCYB11 with the formerly identified chemokines SCYB9 and SCYB10 (Farber JM 1993) revealed striking similarities between the three genes as is shown in *Figure 8*. In all three chemokines, the amino acids encoded by the first exon constitute the signal peptide, and the favourable site of cleavage is predicted to be C-terminal of glycine, the first amino acid of exon 2. In SCYB11 and SCYB10 exon 1 and the signal peptide are of the same size (21 amino acids), while in SCYB9 the amino acids sequence encoding the signal peptide is 1 amino acid longer.

Exon 2 is matching in size in all three chemokines and moreover the intron/exon border of exon 2/intron 3 is found at the same position (the second base of the amino acid triplet coding isoleucine).

The remaining amino acids are splitted to exon 3 and 4. These intron/exon boundaries are less conserved. Especially, exon 4 differs significantly in size in these three chemokines. Of note, for CXCL9 (has the longest exon 4 of all three proteins), a proteolytic processing at the C-terminus is described. The C terminal truncated CXCL9 forms were found to decrease in their ability to induce a Ca^{2+} influx in tumour-infiltrating lymphocytes (Liao F et al. 1995)

	Exon 1	**Intron 1**
huCXCL11	MSVKGMAIALAVILCATVVQ	[585 bp]
huCXCL10	MNQCAILICCLIFLQLSGIQ	[553 bp]
huCXCL9	MKKSGVLFLLGIILLVLIGVQ	[1110bp]

	Exon 2	**Intron 2**
huCXCL11	GFPMFKRGRCLCIGPGVKAVKVADIEKASIMYPSNNCDKIEVI	[99 bp]
huCXCL10	GVPLSRQVRCTCISISNQPVNPRSLEKLEIIPASQFCPRVEII	[235 bp]
huCXCL9	GTPVVRKGRCSCISTNQGTIHLQSLKDLKQFAPSPSCEKIEII	[1253 bp]

	Exon 3	**Intron 3**
huCXCL11	ITLKENKGQRCLNPKSKQARLIIK	[231 bp]
huCXCL10	ATMKKKGEKRCLNPESKAIKNLLKAVSKEM	[436 bp]
huCXCL9	ATLKNGVQTCLNPDSADVKELIKKWEKQ	[1109 bp]

	Exon 4	**Intron 4**
huCXCL11	KVERKNF	... 94 amino acids
huCXCL10	SKRSP	... 98 amino acids
huCXCL9	VSQKKKQKNGKKHQKKKVLKVRKSQRSRQKKTT	.. 125 amino acids

Figure 8: Exon / intron organization of the human chemokines SCYB11, SCYB10 and SCYB9.

The distribution of the encoded amino acids of SCYB11 as compared with SCYB10 and SCYB9 to four exons and the length of introns is shown. The C-terminal proteolytic cleavage of the full length CXCL9 is designated by arrows. Data for SCYB10 were taken from (Luster AD and Ravetch JV 1987). Sequence of human SCYB9 was obtained by sequencing a partial DNA fragment amplified with PCR. Primers were derived from cDNA (GenBank Accession No. X72755).

1.6. Chromosomal localization and arrangement of the genes SCYB11, SCYB10 and SCYB9

To assign the chromosome location for SCYB11, FISH was performed using the two PAC clones (17352 and 17353) as probes mapping to metaphase chromosomes from phytohemagglutinin stimulated normal human lymphocytes. SCYB11 was traced like SCYB9 and SCYB10 on a single locus on the long arm of human chromosome 4 at position 4q21.2 (Erdel M et al. 1998). As described in Introduction, chapter 1.2. Chromosomal localization, the minicluster on human chromosome 4 at position q21.2 is separated from the main CXC cluster by more than 2 Mb (Lee HH and Farber JM 1996, O´Donovan N et al. 1999). In order to refine the mapping of the minicluster and to reveal the arrangement of the orthologous genes in the mouse, two-coloured fibre-FISH experiments were performed.

For fibre-FISH experiments, the human PAC 17352 plasmid DNA and the probes for human SCYB9, SCYB10 and SCYB11 were differentially labelled and hybridised to DNA fibres. The two-colour fibre-FISH experiments were carried out using mechanically stretched chromatin fibres from human blood lymphocytes. To determine the true order of the three chemokines and to calculate their precise distance, a computer-processed composite image of the hybridisations was created. The three chemokines are arranged in the order SCYB9, SCYB10 and SCYB11, in a cluster within a range of 29 kb. The distance between the probes for human SCYB9 to SCYB11, SCYB9 to SCYB10 and SCYB10 to SCYB11 were calculated as 19 kb, 10 kb and 6 kb, respectively. The distance separating SCYB9 ↔ SCYB10 ↔ SCYB11 could be defined as 9 kb and 10 kb (Erdel M et al. submitted). These data are summarized in Figure 9.

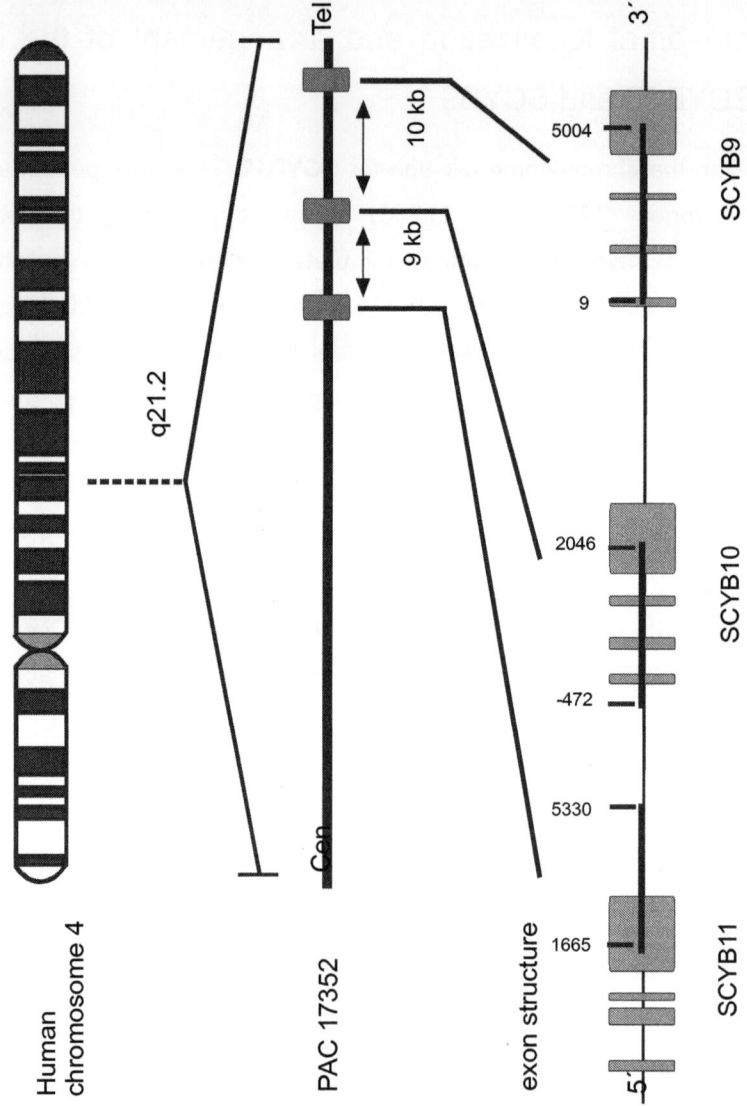

Figure 9: Schematic presentation of CXCL11, CXCL10 and CXCL9 gene arrangement in a minicluster on chromosome 4q21.2.

The Figure combines the result of two different FISH experiments. Mapping the PAC clone to metaphase chromosomes gave the chromosomal location of SCYB11 on human chromosome 4q21.2 (Erdel M et al. 1998). Fibre-FISH experiments showed the arrangement of SCYB11, SCYB10 and SCYB9 in a minicluster on the PAC clone. The three chemokines are clustered in a range of 32 kb on one end of the PAC clone.

The size of the drawn exon (grey boxes) and introns (lines) is schematic and not in scale to the real exon size. The numbers indicate the position of the probes used for fibre-FISH experiments.

1.7. Data of the protein sequence derived from human CXCL11 cDNA

1.7.1. Protein and signal peptide

The reading frame for CXCL11 encodes for a 94 amino acid protein containing a putative 21 amino acid signal sequence characteristic for secretory proteins. A signal peptide is a leader sequence that directs the secreted protein to the ER membrane and is then cleaved off before the mature protein gets exported. The cleavage of the signal peptide underlies specific rules, which have been described by (Heijne G 1982).

The mature protein consists of 73 amino acids as was confirmed by (Tensen CP et al. 1999a). In comparison CXCL10 cDNA encodes for a precursor protein of 98 amino acids with a 21 amino acid signal peptide leading to secretion of a 77 amino acids mature protein. CXCL9 cDNA encodes for a 125 amino acids peptide and contains a signal peptide of 22 amino acids. The mature protein is 103 amino acids long. (See also Introduction, chapter 2.1. Identification of CXCL10 and CXCL9)

1.7.2. Isoelectric point

The mature protein CXCL11 has its isoelectric point at 10.73, as compared with 10.77 for CXCL10, and 11.10 for CXCL9, respectively. This was calculated by the PEPTIDESORT programme from GCG.

1.8. Recombinantly expressed protein

The cDNA encoding the putative mature 73 amino acid CXCL11 protein was modified with the restriction sites KpnI and XhoI and cloned into pET32-a$^+$ as described in Methods, chapter 6.2.4. Cloning into pET32-a expression vector. This resulted in a modified protein that lacked the NH_2-terminal phenylalanine. The recombinant protein was chemotactic for IL-2 selected T memory cells. In contrast, the uncleaved fusion protein containing CXCL11 plus thioredoxin, His-tag and S-tag, as well as the reagent control, had no chemotactic activity over the tested concentration range (Laich A et al. 1998).

In order to obtain the unmodified protein the cDNA of CXCL11 linked to the pET-32a vector, was back-mutated with the *Quick change site-directed mutagenesis kit* (Stratagene) as described in Methods, chapter 6.5. Site-directed mutagenesis.

The recombinantly expressed CXCL11 protein showed to be a potent chemoattractent on IL-2-activated T cells (Laich A et al. 1998). A short description of the chemotactic activity of human CXCL11 is given in Introduction, chapter 2.6.1. Chemotaxis.

1.9. Phylogenetic tree analysis

Comparing nucleotide sequences, the identity of CXCL11 with CXCL9 and CXCL10 is 37.7 % and 44.5 %, respectively. Based on comparison of the amino acid sequences, the identity of CXCL11 with CXCL9 and CXCL10 is 38 % and 32 %, respectively. *Figure 10* shows a dendrogram of the phylogenetic tree (calculated by the PILEUP program from GCG) of all CXC chemokines. The dendrogram underlines the close relationship of CXCL9, CXCL10 and CXCL11 among CXC chemokines. Chemokine sequences available from GenBank are: Accession No X02530 for CXCL10, X72755 for CXCL9, U66096 for CXCL11, M25897 for CXCL4, M26167 for CXCL4V1 (a variant of CXCL4), X53799 for CXCL1, J03561 for CXCL3, X53800 for CXCL2, Y08770 for CXCL6, X78686 for CXCL5, M54995 for CXCL7, Y00787 for CXCL8, AJ002211for CXCL13, and U16752 for CXCL12. The corresponding trivial names are listed in Introduction, *Table1*.

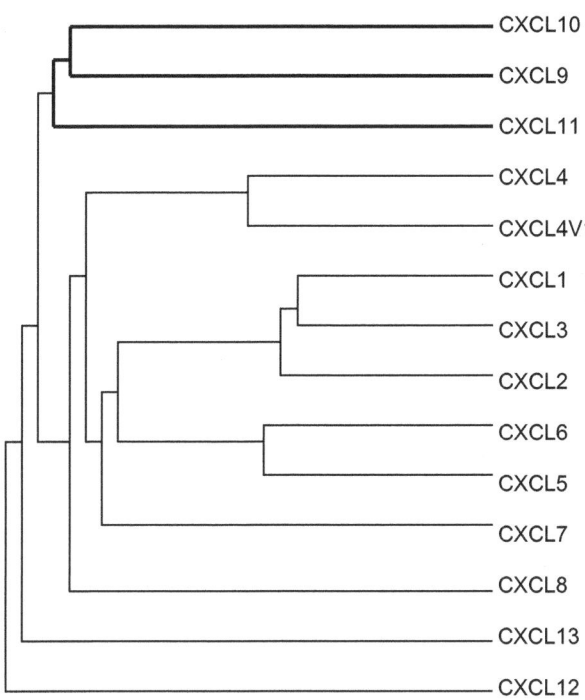

Figure 10: Phylogenetic tree diagram of human CXC chemokines.

The diagram, adopted from Laich A et al. (1999), was calculated with the PILEUP program from GCG. The protein sequences of available CXC chemokines are from GenBank (Accession numbers are listed below).

2. Characterization of murine CXCL11

2.1. Isolation of murine CXCL11 cDNA

Total RNA was isolated from RAW264.7 murine macrophage-like cells treated with 500 U/ml of murine IFN-γ and 1 µg/ml of LPS for 5 hours. cDNA was obtained by standard procedure as described in Methods, chapter 6.3. Reverse transcription.

Primer pair migbse1.prim and migbse2.prim designed from a region of the C-terminus of human CXCL11 were used to amplify a 172 bp product. (Primers are listed in Methods, chapter 7.1.2. List of primer). The PCR product was cloned into the *TA-cloning vector* (Invitrogen) and custom sequenced (Microsynth GmbH).

RACE-PCR was carried out according to the manufactures protocol (*Marathon cDNA Amplification kit*, Clontech) using the *Advantage cDNA polymerase mix*. Primers were mumig1.prim for the 5′-RACE and mumig2.prim for the 3′-RACE. Both primers are listed in Methods, chapter 7.1.2. List of primers.

Two full-length cDNAs (981 bp and 1051 bp / GenBank Accession No. AF136449 and AF178672) were isolated. Both clones are identical except for the polyadenylation signal.

2.2. Analysis of murine CXCL11 cDNA

2.2.1. Characteristic sites found in the murine CXCL11 cDNA

Start codon and Kozak sequence

The sequence flanking the start codon of murine CXCL11 GAG**ATG**A (see *Figure 11*) is less commonly used among mammalian mRNAs but is operative in about 7 % of the sequences analysed. Although this site lacks the optimal sequence, the purine in position -3, which was shown to be necessary for the initiation, is still found. (Kozak M 1987). In comparison, the Kozak sequence of human CXCL11 is AAC**ATG**A, a sequence which ranks higher in the efficiency to initiate the translation.

Polyadenylation signals

Two full-length cDNAs (981 bp and 1051 bp) identical except for the polyadenylation signals used were obtained. The shorter 981 bp clone has the classical polyadenylation signal AATAAA positioned 29 bp before the 3´ end. The longer clone (1051 bp) uses the rare polyadenylation signal AATATA, which is found 14 bp before the 3´end. Many genes have been described to contain multiple poly-A$^+$ sites within the 3´UTR. The regulation of polyadenylation is supposed to play an important role in gene expression, since it was described by (Gilbert-Edwalds G et al. 1997) that the poly-A site strength can regulate the amount of cytoplasmic RNA by influencing the mRNA-stability.

This finding is in agreement with data derived from the human CXCL11 cDNAs. As mentioned in Results, chapter 1.2.1. Characteristic sites of human CXCL11 cDNA, human CXCL11 cDNAs isolated from various human cell types were also found to use different polyadenylation sites (Laich A et al. 1998).

AREs

Like the 3´ UTR of human CXCL11, the murine CXCL11 3´ UTR also contains T-rich domains and the pentanucleotide ATTTA characteristic for AT-rich elements (AREs). AREs can function as potent mRNA destabilizing elements and are responsible for selective and rapid mRNA degradation (Chen CYA and Shyu AB 1995).

2.3. Isolation of the genomic murine *Scyb11* sequence

Genomic DNA was isolated from RAW264.7 cells with the *Blood and Cell Culture DNA kit* (Qiagen). With the primer pair migbse1.prim and migbse2.prim (see

Methods, chapter 7.1.2. List of primers) directed to flanking sequences of the cDNA PCR fragment, a 215 bp genomic DNA fragment was amplified which contained a partial sequence of exon 2 and exon 3 covering intron 2. Using these conditions, mouse BAC libraries were screened by custom service (Genome Systems, St. Louis, Missouri) but no positive clones could be isolated.

Therefore we used the Genome Walking strategy (*Mouse Genome Walking kit* and *Advantage-GC Genomic Polymerase Mix*) to obtain genomic sequences of murine *Scyb11*. A detailed description of the Genome Walking strategy is found in Methods, chapter 7.3. Genome Walking). In summary, we obtained 4631 bp of the genomic sequence of murine *Scyb11* including the 5′and 3′ flanking regions with six primer walking reactions.

From this sequence 447 bp belong to the 5′ flanking region and about 1000 bp to the region behind the polyadenylation site. The complete sequence is shown in *Figure 11*.

A 1300 bp clone obtained by Genome Walking and containing intron 1 and exon 2 was then used for screening a BAC mouse library (Genome Systems). One positive BAC clone (BAC 22256) was isolated. This clone was used in addition to genome walking to analyse the genomic sequence of murine *Scyb11*. The genomic sequence was submitted to GenBank (Accession No. AF167354).

```
-447   AAAAAAAAAAATAGACACAATGTACAGCTATGGGGAGAGTGTTTCAGGCATGAAATTGGAAGGAAAAAAAAAAGTAAAGAT
                                                            NF-AT           GAGA-1

-367   AGATGAAGGTCACCTGGTATGTATAATATATGCCTTATCCATATATGTGTGGTTATGTGAGGGAGGCAGGATGAGCTGCC
                                          GATA-1

-287   TGGAACTGGGACCATCTTCCTGAGTTGGTGGGACTCTGCCCAGAATCCCTACACAATCAAAGCATTTCTAGGAAAAGCCA
                                                                              NF-κB

-207   CCTGCTGAGCAGCTGCTGAGTGCTTTCACCTTCCAGTGGCTTCTTAACTCCAGCAGAGGGGACAGTCACAGCGCTGACTT

-127   AAGGACAAAAGAGAAACTCCAGGAGGCAAGAAAGCTACGTGAGTCAAGGAGGGGAATTCCTGATACTGCCTGAAGATTGC
           IRF-1 / ISRE                             AP-1        NF-κB

-47    TGGTCTATAAATGCTCCTCAGACTCCTCAGGTTCAGCCTTCCTGCCTGCCGTTGCTCTCTGCAAAGAGAGATCTCCAAAG
            TATA-box                                      +1

 33    CCCAGGCAGAGAGCTGCAGCGGCTGCTGAGATGAACAGGAAGGTCACAGCCATAGCCCTGGCTGCGATCATCTGGGCCAC
                                       M  N  R  K  V  T  A  I  A  L  A  A  I  I  W  A  T

113    AGCTGCTCAAGGTATTTGGTGCCCGTAGCTTCTGAGTCTGTCTGTTCCTTGTGTTACTTTTCAAATATCTTTTTCTCTAA
```

```
                A   A   Q
193   AATATACAGTTTTAAAATTTTACTTTATTTCACATATTAGAAGTTCTAAGGGGAGGGTATAGGGAACTTTCGGGATAGCA
273   TTTGAAATGTATATAAAGAAAATATCTAATAAAAAATAAATAATTAAAAAAAGAAGTTCTAGCAATGGCACAGCAAATGT
353   TGGAAATCCTTAAAGAAAATGATCAGTTTATGGATTCATTTTCTTTCTTTCCTTCTTCCTTCCTTCCTTCCTTCCTTCCT
433   TCCTTCCTTCCTTCCTTCCTTTCTTTCTTTCTTTCTTTCTTTCTCTCTTTCTTTCTCTCCTTCTCTCTTTCTCTCTCTCT
513   TCCCTCTCTTCCTCTCTTCCTCTCTTCCTCTCTTTCTTTCTCTCTTTCTCTCTTTCTCTCTTTCTCTCTTTCTTTCTTTC
593   CTGGTTTTTTCAAGACAGGGTTTCTCTGTGTAGCCCTGGCTGTCCTGGAACTCACTCTGTAGACCAGGCTGGCCTCAAAC
673   TCAGAAATCCGCCTGCCTCTGCCTCCCAAGTGCTGGGATAAAAGGCGCGCACCACCACACCTGGCGATTTGTATTTCAAA
753   TAAACCACAGATATTATGGTCAGAGCAACTTACAAATATTAGGCAGTAAACAATGCCATTGTATTCCTCCACAGTTGTTA
833   GTACTGGGATTAAAGGCGTGCGCCACCCCTGCCCAATTTCTTCATTTTCTGACAATTATCCAGTCCTCAATGCCTGTTCA
913   GAGAATCTTATGTGGGATTATGCTGGTATTCTGAAAAAATTAATGTTTTAACCAGGAGACTGCTAATTTGTTATGACCAA
993   TACTTTCAGAATAGAGAAAAGGAAATTTCTCTCTGGGGCAATGGTCATAAAAATGTCATACGTGCTTGATCAATATGTCA
1073  CTTGAGGGCAAGAGTGACTTAAAGGTAGTGTGGATACTGACAATGCTCCACAAGCTCTTCCCAAAGAATATTGTTTCTAA
1153  ATAGAAGCATTATTCACATGTCCCATGACTGAACCTGGAAGTGTTTCTCCTGTGAGTTGATGGTTCTTACGCGATTATCA
1233  CAGCAGACCTGGGCTAAGCCAGATATGAAGTTAATGTGACAAGCCAAGCCATTATTACAACTCTTGCTGCTCTTATGAAA
1313  TAATGAACCTTTGAGGTTTCCCTGGGAGCATCTGGAAGCTTTAAAGACAGTTTCAGCTGTGGGAGACAACATGATTCATA
1393  ATACTTAGTCTTAATCTAGAATTTGAACTGGGAAGACAAAGATCAAAGAAATTATCAACTATTTGCTCATTTAGTAAAGA
1473  ACAGATCACCAGCGACTGTGAAAGACGCTTGTATACCCATTCCACCAGTCATAAAATAATTCCAAATAAATAGCCACTTT
1553  GTTCTCTGGGTTGCTGTATACTGTGTAGGTGTTATTTAAAGTAATCAAGAGCCGGTCTCATAGCATACTCATACTGTAAT
1633  ATAACTTCAGCACTTAGGAGGGTGAGCTGAGTGAGGTAGGATAATGCCAAGATGGGGGGAGGGGGCTGCTTTGTAGTGAG
1713  TGCTTCAAGTTCAAAGTCATCCTGGGCTTTGTGGTGAGTTGGAAGCAAACCTGGTCCAAATAGCAAGTGAGTCCTGTCTG
1793  CAACCTAAATTAAATAATTAACAAAAATTAAGGAAGGAAATCATCAAGGATACAGCAAATTAGCCTAATGCAGAGAGATT
1873  CAAAAACTTAATTTCAGTCTGCACAGTTGAGATTAACAAATGCGTCTGCCATCCACTTCACAGCCCTGACTAACCAACAC
1953  TGTGGTCTGTCCCAG**GCTTCCTTATGTTCAAACAGGGGCGCTGTCTTTGCATCGGCCCCGGGATGAAAGCCGTCAAAATG**
                  G   F   L   M   F   K   Q   G   R   C   L   C   I   G   P   G   M   K   A   V   K   M
2033  **GCAGAGATCGAGAAAGCTTCTGTAATTTACCCGAGTAACGGCTGCGACAAAGTTGAAGTGAT**GTATGTGCTGGAGGTGAC
      A   E   I   E   K   A   S   V   I   Y   P   S   N   G   C   D   K   V   E   V   I
2113  AATGGTATGGGTGCTTTTGTTTGGTTGATGTTTTCCCACCAAAGTTTAAGACTCTTTTGTGTCTCCCTTACCAG**TGTTAC**
                                                                                      V   T
2193  **TATGAAGGCTCATAAACGACAAAGGTGCCTGGACCCCAGATCCAAGCAAGCTCGCCTCATAATGCAG**GTAGGTTGCCAGT
       M   K   A   H   K   R   Q   R   C   L   D   P   R   S   K   Q   A   R   L   I   M   Q
2273  CGGCCAGGTCGGAAAGTGCTTTACCCACGAGAGTGCTGGAACACAGAGAACAGGCGACTGCCGGAAGACCCCATTACCAT
2353  CCTAACAGAAGCACCCAGTTAAGGGGTCCTGGGTTAAAACCTGGCCACATCCTTACCCCTCCGCGTTGTTTTTACAGGTCA
2433  GCTCTTAATTACTGAGGAAACGAAACAACCCAGTAAGTAAAACTCTTCATTTTCTCATTACAG**GCAATAGAAAAAAAGAA**
                                                                        A   I   E   K   K   N
2513  **TTTTTTAAGGCGTCAAAACATGTGACATCCTGGGAACGTCTGACTGTGAGCCCTCCAATAAGAACTCTGTGCCAGGAACC**
       F   L   R   R   Q   N   M   *
2593  **TGACCCTCTGCTGTCTTGGAACATGCAGCCACGTATTACCAGGCTGCAGAACTTTCTAGAAGGTCCGATACATCTAAACT**
2673  **GTTCTACTTGGCTATGAAAAATATTTGTCTCTAAAAGTCATGTGCACACTCCACGCTACCTTCTGTGGTTACAGTGGATG**
2753  **CATTGTTACTGCAATCCGGACCAGTGCTGGATTCAAAAGCATCTCTGTGTGTAGTAAAACATTCCTCAAAGAATTGTTCA**
2833  **TGCAAATAAACATTCCTTTCCCCAAATATCACGAGGCACACGAACATCTAGGAAGACATTTCCACATTTGTCTTGTTTG**
2913  **TTCATTTAAAAAGACTACGATTCATTTCTGCGTTGTANAAACTAGTAAGAACACTACTGTTTGTTTCCTAGCTAGTCACA**
2993  **CTGGCTTCCCCCTGAGGCCTTCTAAGGGGTTAAGATGTGTATTTCCTGTACGTCTGGTTTTATCAGTGACAATAACAAGG**
```

```
3073  ATAGATTTTTAAAAATAAATTGGTTCTGTTCACCAAAGAAAAATGTTGAAAAAAAAATCTGTGCACCTCTTTCAGTCTGTT
                    poly A site
3153  TCCTGTGAGTCTGCCTTTGAGAAAAATATATAAATATGTACTTTGTTCTTTTCCTTGGTCATACTGTGAATGAATGGTAG
                          poly A site
3233  GGATGGCTGGCTCTGTCTCTCCTTGAAAAGAATAAGAATTGTGTTTCTCTAGTAAGCTATTATAACACTTATTAAATCAT
3313  CACCAACTACATGCTCTCTGGACATTGAGATGCCTTTAGATTTTGTTTTGTTTTGTTTTGTTTTTTTAGAGCTACACAAGT
3393  TTTTGTCAGAATTCTTTAGAAACATACACGCCTTTAATCCCAGCACTTGGGAGGCAGAGGCAGGCGGATCTCTGTGAGGT
3473  CCAGGCCAGACTGGTCTTTCAGAACAGTCAGGGCTACACAAAATTTTAAAATAGAAAGGAATATACTTTAGTGAGGAGGA
3553  GCTGAAGATGAGAAAAAAATATGATAAAAAGGTACTGTTAAAAATTTCAATAAAAAAAATTACCTAGGTGTGGTGGTATA
3633  CACCTTAATTTCAGCACTTGAAAGGCAGAGGCAGGAGGATCTCTTGAGTTCAAGGCCAACCTGGTCTACAGACCAGGAGT
3713  TTCAGGACAGCCAGGGCTACACAGAGAAACCCTATCTTAAAGTAAAGAAAAAAAGAAATGCCCAAATAAAATAAAATAAA
3793  ATAAAGAAAGGGAGGAAGGAAGGAAGAAAAGAAAAAGAAATGTACTTCGATAGTAGTCATAAAGGAATCTAATCAACTTC
3873  ACTTAGGATTGAAGAGACTCTCCCTGGCTGCCCCACCCCAGCCCCTTTCATGTCTGTTAAATCTCTCCTATTGTGACTTT
3953  CTGAGCTGCGCCAAAAGGGGAAAGCAAAGGGAGATTTCCTGCCAAGCACAGCAAAGCCCCAGCCAGGCTGTGTGTACTCA
4033  GACTTTGCACCTCAGAGAGGGCACAGCGACTGTCATGGAGAAACCTGAAATAGCAGACCAGCCCGGGCCGTCGACCACGC
4113  GTGCCCTATAGTGAGTCGTATTACACCAGCCCGGGCGTCGACCACGCGTGCCCTATAGTGAGTCGTATTACT
```

Figure 11: Genomic sequence of murine *Scyb11.*

Numbers on the left are relative to the putative transcription initiation site (+1). Underlined sequences correspond to known transcription factor binding sites. The cDNA is present in bold letters. The polyadenylation signals were indicated by underlining. The deduced amino acid sequence is written below the cDNA.

2.4. Analysis of the promoter region / comparison to the human promoter

2.4.1. Computer assisted analysis of transcription factor binding sites

The sequence up to -447 was analysed with MatInspector (http://genomatrix.gsf.de), a program to detect transcription factor binding sites. The same subset of matrices for analysis of the human CXCL11 promoter region was used. The matrices obtained from TRANSFAC (http://transfac.gbf.de.TRANSFAC) are listed in Appendix, 1. List of regulatory elements found in the promoter region.

The murine *Scyb11* promoter contains one TATA box but no CAAT box. Furthermore, two NF-κB sites and one interferon-responsive element (ISRE) were found. Functional promoter analysis of murine *Scyb9* and *Scyb10* suggested that the most important regulatory elements are close to the transcription start site and that the interferon-regulatory-site and the NF-κB sites have synergistic effects (Ohmori Y and Hamilton TA 1993, Ohmori Y et al. 1997). This could be also suggested for murine *Scyb11* and awaits further analysis.

Comparing the transcription factor binding sites of murine *Scyb11* with murine *Scyb10* and murine *Scyb9* shows that like *Scyb10*, also *Scyb11* contains two NF-κB sites. The palindromic element γRE-1 essential for the IFN-γ response in murine *Scyb9* (Wong P et al. 1994) could not be found in murine *Scyb11*.

2.4.2. Sequence comparison to human SCYB11

Sequence alignment of the 5′ flanking region of human SCYB11 and murine *Scyb11* shows that about 150 bp are homologous (shown in *Figure 12*). Among several important binding sites identified in this region the TATA-box and binding sites for regulatory elements, like the ISRE, one NF-κB site and the AP-1 site are conserved. Interestingly, the relative position and spacing of these elements and also the distance to the site of transcription initiation are well conserved. It can be speculated that the distance and range of regulatory elements can influence the strength of transcription as was shown for the murine *Scyb9* (Ohmori Y et al. 1997). However, the synergistic or antagonistic effects of regulatory elements in the human and mouse SCYB11 promoter remain to be proved by functional analysis and by site-specific mutations.

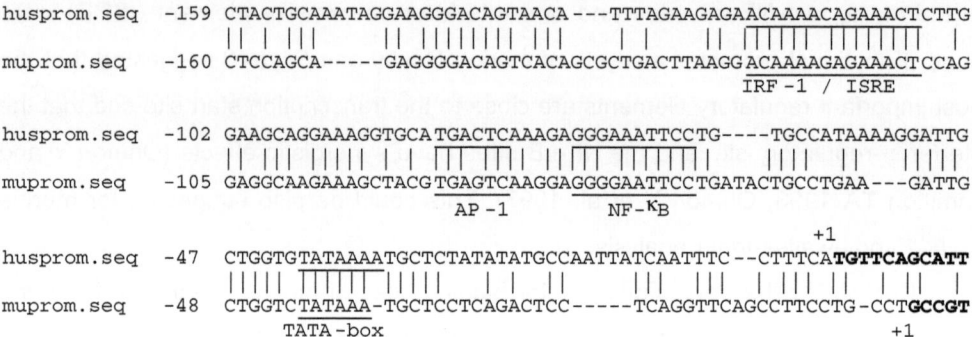

Figure 12: Alignment of murine and human SCYB11 promoter

150 bp of the upstream DNA sequence of human SCYB11 (husprom.seq) and murine *Scyb11* (muprom.seq) (analysed with MatInspector) were aligned and conserved putative enhancer elements (underlined) were identified. Numbers refer to the determined transcription start of human SCYB11 and the hypothetical transcription start of murine *Scyb11*.

2.5. Comparison of the genomic structure of murine and human SCYB11

Murine *Scyb11* is organized in 4 exons like its human counterpart. Furthermore, the distribution of the amino acids over the 4 exons is highly similar in both genes and in both human and mouse SCYB11, all exon/intron splice junctions follow the GT/AG rule. However, the murine *Scyb11* gene is considerably longer than human SCYB11 due to its intron 1 sequence being ~1800 bp. This intron contains a 201 bp stretch of irregularly repeated TTTC, CTTC, TTCC, and TC motifs. These simple repeats may represent sequences of cryptic simplicity (Seffert W et al. 1998). Repetitive simple sequences occur found in many eukaryotic genomes. It is proposed that they arose by a common mechanism, namely slippage replication and unequal crossing over, and that they might have no general function (Tautz D and Renz M 1984).

The genomic murine *Scyb10* sequence (GenBank Accession No. P17515) shows high similarities in the intron/exon organization (Vanguri P and Farber JM 1990), (data not shown). A comparison with murine *Scyb9* was not possible since this genomic sequence (cDNA sequence first published in 1990) is still not available from GenBank.

	Exon 1	**Intron 1**
muCXCL11	MNRKVTAIALAAIIWATAAQ	[1845 bp]
huCXCL11	MSVKGMAIALAVILCATVVQ	[585 bp]

	Exon 2	**Intron 2**
muCXCL11	GFLMFKQGRCLCIGPGMKAVKMAEIEKASVIYPSNGCDKVEVI	[93 bp]
huCXCL11	GFPMFKRGRCLCIGPGVKAVKVADIEKASIMYPSNNCDKIEVI	[99 bp]

	Exon 3	**Intron 3**
muCXCL11	VTMKAHKRQRCLDPRSKQARLIMQ	[237 bp]
huCXCL11	ITLKENKGQRCLNPKSKQARLIIK	[231 bp]

	Exon 4	
muCXCL11	AIEKKNFLRRQNM	... 100 amino acids
huCXCL11	KVERKNF	... 94 amino acids

Figure 13: Comparison of the exon/intron organization of murine *Scyb11* and human homologue. Amino acid sequences, the nucleotide length and the size of the three introns are presented.

2.6. Chromosomal localization and gene arrangement of *Scyb11*, *Scyb10* and *Scyb9*

The chromosomal mapping of murine *Scyb11* was carried out by FISH experiments using the BAC clone as a probe and metaphase chromosomes from two different cell lines (Balb/c mice (3T3) and dermal fibroblasts). Chromosomal mapping localizes *Scyb11* to chromosome 5 at position 5E3 (Meyer M et al. 2000). This location is orthologous to the human chromosome localization 4q21.

Previous work showed that the murine genes *Scyb9* and *Scyb10* are also located on mouse chromosome 5 in a position orthologous to human SCYB9 and SCYB10 genes (Modi WS et al. 1998). In order to reveal the arrangement of the orthologous genes in the mouse, we performed two-colour fibre-FISH experiments using mechanically stretched chromatin fibres from agarose embedded cells. The three chemokine genes are situated in a similar configuration in the two species. The chemokines are arranged in the order *Scyb9* ↔ *Scyb10* ↔ *Scyb11*. After correction of these measurements according to the relative position of the chemokine probes, all 3 genes cluster in a range of 32 kb in mouse. The distance separating the genes *Scyb9*, *Scyb10* and *Scyb11* could be defined as 9 kb and 14 kb (Erdel M et al. submitted). A schematic presentation of the gene arrangement is given in *Figure 14*.

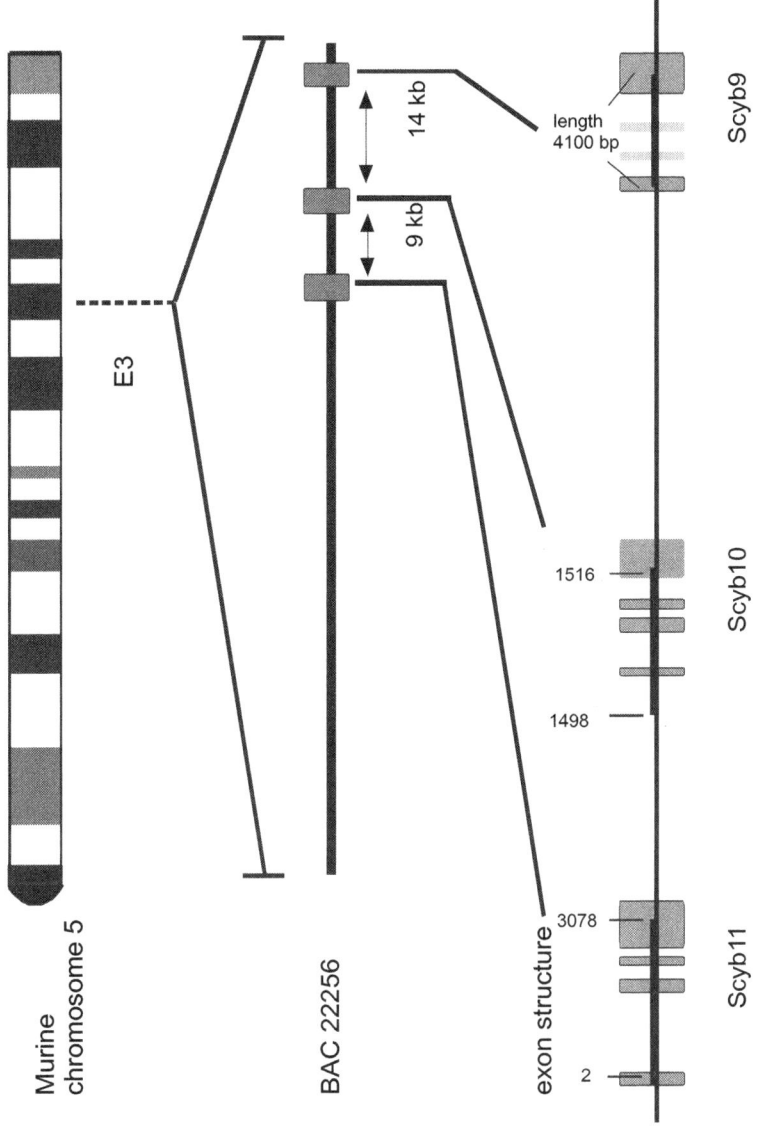

Figure 14: Schematic presentation of murine *Scyb11*, *Scyb10* and *Scyb9* arrangement in a minicluster on chromosome 5E3.

The Figure combines the results of two different FISH experiments. Mapping the BAC 22256 clone to metaphase chromosome gave the chromosomal location of *Scyb11* on mouse chromosome 5E3 (Meyer M et al. 2000). Fibre-FISH experiments revealed the arrangement of *Scyb11*, *Scyb10* and *Scyb9* in a minicluster on the BAC clone. The three chemokines are clustered in a range of 29 kb on one end of the BAC clone. The size of the drawn exon (grey boxes) and introns (lines) is schematic and not true to scale. The numbers indicate the positions of the probes used for fibre-FISH.

2.7. Data of the protein sequence derived from murine CXCL11 cDNA

2.7.1. Protein and signal peptide

The reading frame deduced from the murine CXCL11 encodes a 100 amino acid protein. The 21 amino acids at the N-terminus are predicted to encode a signal peptide, leaving a mature secretion protein of 79 amino acids (von Heijne G 1983).

In comparison murine CXCL10 and CXCL9 mRNAs encode a 98 and 126 amino acid immature proteins and both are predicted to encode also a signal peptide of 21 amino acids (Vanguri P and Farber JM 1990, Farber JM 1990). Recent work showed that mature murine CXCL11 recombinantly expressed in Drosophila S2 cells starts with the FPMFK sequence as predicted (Hensbergen PJ et al. in preparation).

2.7.2. Molecular mass

The calculated molecular masses are 11.265 Da for immature and 9.113 Da for mature murine CXCL11. Considering the two disulphide bounds the Mr is 9010. For comparison, molecular masses deduced for the mature proteins of muCXCL9 are 12.193 Da (Farber JM. 1990) and for CXCL10 8.700 Da (Vanguri P and Farber JM 1990, Ohmori Y and Hamilton TA. 1990).

2.7.3. Sequence identity of human and murine CXCL11

The identity of immature human and mouse CXCL11 amino acid sequence is 68 %. Nucleotide sequence of human and mouse CXCL11 share 63 % identity. Homology to murine CXCL9 and CXCL10 is 33.3 % and 26.0 % amino acid identity, respectively, as was calculated for the immature proteins.

2.7.4. Isoelelectric point

The respective isoelectric points are calculated to be 11.06 for the immature protein and 10.86 for the mature protein.

2.8. Phylogenetic tree analysis

Phylogenetic tree analysis of ten available mouse CXC chemokines indicates that the murine chemokines CXCL11, CXCL9 and CXCL10 share an individual branch of the evolutionary tree. (shown in *Figure 15*). The diagram was calculated by the PILEUP program from GCG using immature protein sequences available from GenBank. CXCL1 (Accession No. P12850), CXCL2 (P10889), CXCL5 (AAC52238), CXCL9 (P18340), CXCL10 (P17515), CXCL11 (AF136449), CXCL12 (P40224), CXCL13 (AAC34603), CXCL 14 (AAD34157) and CXCL15 (AAD38079). The corresponding trivial names are listed in Introduction, *Table 1*.

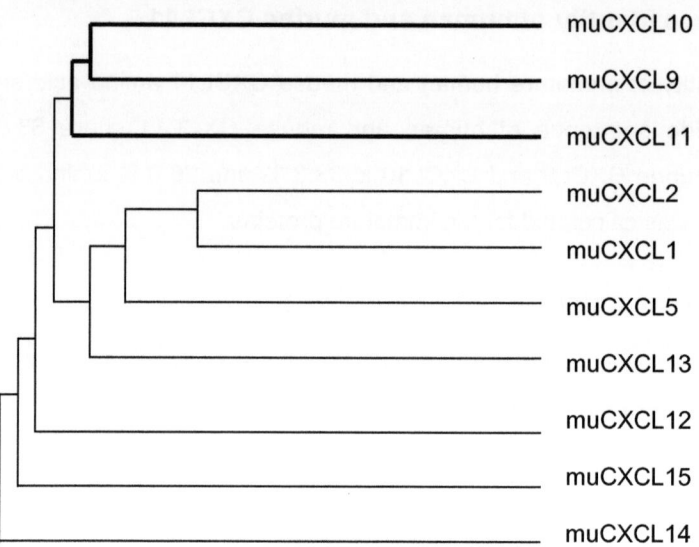

Figure 15: Phylogenetic tree diagram of murine CXC chemokines.

The diagram (adopted from Meyer M et al. 2000) was calculated by PILEUP using immature protein sequences (available from GenBank). Accession numbers are listed above.

IV. Discussion

In the last few years, the chemokine field extended very fast. One problem the field faced following the rapid pace of chemokine discovery is that several groups reported the same cDNA molecule simultaneously under different names. This also happened with human CXCL11 alias βR1, H174, SCYB9B, I-TAC, and IP-9. Although some research results overlap, many additional information became available, which makes it possible to discuss findings on human and murine CXCL11 in a broad context.

Human CXCL11 was characterized by different groups: The first partial cDNA was cloned from IFN-γ-stimulated astrocytoma cells line (Rani MSR et al. 1996) and a strong up-regulation of this cDNA upon IFN-γ and IFN-β stimulation was shown. However, due to sequence errors the chemokine nature of this partial cDNA was not revealed at first.

Next, a partial cDNA sequence, was published (Jacobs KA et al. 1997), which was isolated from activated PBMC by a method specifically developed to isolate signal peptide containing sequences. In 1998, the complete cDNA isolated from cytokine-activated human astrocytoma cells was published and the chemokine nature of the synthetic protein deduced from the cDNA was confirmed (Cole KE et al. 1998). In addition, it was shown that this novel chemokine activates cells via the CXCR3 receptor, the common receptor for CXCL9 and CXCL10, which is expressed on Th1 memory cells (Loetscher ML et al. 1996). Also, tissue-specific distribution and IFN-induction in astrocytes and monocytes were investigated.

Our own group isolated a full-length CXCL11 cDNA sequence from IFN-γ-treated human myelomonocytic cells and characterized its genomic structure using the PAC clone used before for chromosome localization (Erdel M et al. 1998). We also investigated the mRNA expression of CXCL11 upon various IFNs in THP-1 cells and the expression pattern in various human cell lines including endothelial cells, fibroblasts and primary monocytes. The recombinant protein was chemotactic for IL-2-treated T memory cells (see Results, <u>chapter 1.7. Recombinantly expressed protein</u>).

The native mature protein (initially termed IP-9) was isolated from IFN-γ-treated human keratinocytes. This amino acid sequence was used to clone a full-length cDNA from human kerationcytes, which was also recombinantly expressed and active via CXCR3 receptor. Furthermore, differential expression in various skin diseases was shown (Tensen CP et al. 1999a). In another paper the same group published a genomic sequence including 960 bp of the 5´ region and regulatory elements such as the transcription start site and regulatory binding motifs were putatively assigned (Tensen CP et al. 1999b).

The comparison of these data allows several conclusions: CXCL11 mRNA from different cell sources varies in length at the 3´ terminus because of the usage of different polyadenylation sites. An alignment of these cDNAs shows a polymorphism of CXCL11 in THP-1 cells. Since a detailed analysis of CXCL11 mRNA expression in various cell types is available, these data can be set in relation to the structural and functional promoter analysis of huCXCL11 described below.

Only recently, our group described the homologous murine sequence muCXCL11. The cDNA was isolated from IFN-γ/LPS-stimulated RAW264.7 mouse macrophage-like cells (Meyer M et al. 2000). We could also identify its genomic organization and chromosome localization. In the same year, the cDNA was also cloned from a cDNA library made from lung of adrenalectomized and LPS-treated mice (Widney DP et al. 2000). Again the cDNAs vary in their length at the 3´-terminus. The cDNA sequences of human and murine CXCL11 were compared and shown to be highly similar in their exon/intron organization.

A database search reveals the high homology of CXCL11 with the CXC-chemokines CXCL10 and CXCL9. Both chemokines have been identified several years before and are now well characterized (Luster AD et al. 1985, Farber JM. 1990). Here we compare the amino acid sequence and show that the three related chemokines form an individual branch on the phylogenetic tree. Moreover, the chemokines are linked in a minicluster with identical arrangement in man and mouse.

Thus a comparison of the related chemokines CXCL9, CXCL10 and CXCL11 allows a view on the evolutionary development of this chemokine subfamily.

Gene regulation

Human CXCL11 mRNA expression patterns from different cell types were identified by Northern blot analysis (Laich A et al. 1999) and quantitative PCR (Cole KE et al. 1998). In general, it is indicated that various stimuli may activate mRNA expression in a cell specific way. Comparing these data and the structural and functional promoter analysis gives an insight into CXCL11 gene regulation.

The mRNA expression in all cell types is strongly induced by IFN-γ (Laich A et al. 1999). IFN-β as a single stimulus also shows a relevant induction as was demonstrated in the human astrocytoma cell-line CRT, whereas IFN-α is only a weak stimulus (Rani MRS et al. 1996).IL-1β, IL-4, IL-6, IL-13, TNF-α and LPS as single stimuli could not upregulate the mRNA production as was seen on Northern blots. In some cell lines (like THP-1 cells and HepG2), LPS enhanced the IFN-γ-induced CXCL11 mRNA levels (Laich A et al. 1999).

A computer-assisted inspection of the 5´ region flanking the CXCL11 coding region identified four IFN– responsive elements (GAS, ISRE and two IRF sites) in the promoter region between -105 and -404. Furthermore, one NF-κB site at position -65 and two NF-IL6 sites (positions -178 and -364) were obtained. A functional promoter analysis was carried out with HepG2 cells transfected with various CXCL11 promoter–luciferase reporter gene constructs. This demonstrated that a promoter fragment up to -301, containing the ISGF-3, the NF-κB and the GAS transcription factor-binding site shows a very strong induction upon IFN-γ and also a good induction upon IFN-β, whereas IFN-α was only a weak stimulus.

IL-1β and LPS as a single stimulus showed no effects on the promoter and LPS could not potentate the effect of IFN-γ, which contradicts our observations made with THP-1 cells using Northern blot analysis. This discrepancy may be explained by an possible alteration of mRNA stability in response to LPS.

TNF-α as a single stimulus showed a moderate induction in the -301 bp fragment but the effect of TNF-α could be enhanced by IL-1β in the -409 bp fragment suggesting that cooperative interactions between the NF-κB site and more distant sites are possible.

Experimental findings demonstrate the possibility of additional regulatory elements distal to the -409 promoter fragment, which are functionally distinct. A negative element between -1520 and -2601 suppresses response to IFN-γ, while a positive element between -2601 and -3433 enhances the response to IFN-γ. Further work will show whether these elements are functional and which transcription regulatory elements are involved.

The murine *Scyb11* promoter is known up to base -447. A computer assisted inspection revealed several transcription regulatory binding sites like two NF-κB sites (at position -68 and -208), one ISRE site (at position -110) and one AP-1 site (at position -81). In comparison, the human SCYB11 promoter contains only one NF-κB site, which is analogous to murine NF-κB(1).

Over 190 bp, the 5´ flanking region between the human and mouse genes are 69.6 % identical. Within this promoter section, several conserved regulatory elements including the ISRE and NF-κB site are found. Furthermore, the TATA sequence necessary for binding of the general transcription factors, and thus important for initiation of transcription by RNA polymerase II, is conserved. The relative position and spacing of these elements and also the distance to the transcription start site in human and mouse SCYB11 is identical suggesting that these conserved elements have identical function in both species. In order to prove functionality of these putative transcription factor binding sites, careful studies of the murine promoter e.g. site-directed mutagenisis will be necessary.

Regulatory elements on RNA level

CXCL11 cDNAs isolated from different cell types were found to use different polyadenylation signals. A 995 bp long cDNA clone isolated from activated PBMC (Jacobs KA et al. 1997) uses the TATAAG-signal at position 1791, according to the SCYB11 DNA shown in *Figure 6*. Furthermore, a 1371 bp cDNA clone (GenBank Accession No. AF030514) isolated from human fetal astrocytes stimulated with TNF-α in combination with IFN-γ and IL-1β which uses the rare polyadenylation signal AATACA, at position 2261 of the SCYB11 DNA was published (Cole KE et al. 1998). The CXCL11 cDNA isolated from THP-1 cells (1445 bp in length) was found to use the classical AATAAA polyadenylation signal at position 2358.

Furthermore, several putative polyadenylation signals can be identified within the 3´ UTR of the SCYB11 cDNA (detailed list in Laich A et al. 1999). It remains to be seen whether some of these signals are functional in addition to the already identified polyadenylation signals.

Isolation of the murine homologue muCXCL11 from RAW264.7 cells brought up two cDNAs identical except for the polyadenylation signal used. The classical polyadenylation signal AATAAA was obtained on the 981 bp clone (29 bp before the 3´end) and the rare polyadenylation signal AATATA on the 1051 bp clone (found 14 bp before the 3´end). In addition, a search of glucocorticoid-attenuated response genes identified two murine CXCL11 cDNA clones isolated from lung of adrenalectomized and LPS treated mice. One of the clones was described to use the rare polyadenylation signal AATATA like the 1051 bp clone isolated from RAW246.7 cells. The other clone terminates 567 bp later (at position 3754 on the genomic DNA shown in *Figure 11*). Interestingly, no polyadenylation site was described for this clone (Widney DP et al. 2000).

Although most eukaryotic genes are described to contain only a single polyadenylation signal, a growing number of genes are known that have two or more polyadenylation sites (Edwalds-Gilbert G et al. 1997). The so-called tandem polyadenylation sites are arranged one behind the other within the 3′ UTR of a single 3′ terminal exon. Of note, some of the genes with tandem polyadenylation sites are regulated by differential use of these sites, for example, during cell cycle or in a tissue-specific pattern (Edwalds-Gilbert G et al. 1997).

Another common finding in the 3′ UTR region of man and mouse CXCL11 cDNA are AREs. Several AT-rich stretches and T-rich domains, which may determine mRNA stability, can be detected in both cDNAs. These elements are found in the 3′ UTR region of many mRNAs encoding cytokines and nuclear transcription factors (Chen CYA and Shyu AB 1995).

Thus, CXCL11 possibly adds a new member to the group of genes, which can control gene expression on the mRNA level by degradation and variable 3′ UTR length.

Sequence comparison

The overall structure of human and mouse SCYB11 are highly similar. Both genes comprise four exons, of which the first three are identical with regard to exon size and the location of exon-intron splice junctions. Size differences were only found in exon 4. Murine CXCL11 has six additional residues at the carboxyl terminus not present in the human protein.

The 73 aligned residues of the predicted mature peptides are 71 % identical and 93 % similar, whereas the signal sequences are 57 % identical and 63 % similar. The predicted mature murine CXCL11 protein is found to have much greater similarity to human CXCL11 than to the most closely related murine chemokines muCXCL10 and muCXCL9 (Widney DP et al. 2000).

The transcription start sites of the human gene have been characterized by primer extension. Although the transcription start site of the mouse gene was not determined by an experimental approach it is supposed to be next to the location of the start site in the human gene. Race-PCR identified two cDNA clones with an identical 5´ end 36 nucleotides before the TATA-box as compared to 34 nucleotides proved in the human gene.

Repetitive elements

Beside these striking similarities, two sequence deviations are found in murine *Scyb11*. The intron 1 of murine *Scyb11* which differs most in the comparison of human and murine *Scyb11* intron/exon structure, contains a 201 bp stretch of irregularly repeated TTC, CTTC, TTCC, and TC motifs. These simple repeats may represent sequences of high cryptic simplicity, which are known to show a particularly fast evolutionary turnover (reviewed by Tautz D and Schlötterer C 1994).

A mouse B1 repetitive sequence is reported in the 3´ UTR of the murine CXCL11 cDNA (Widney DP et al. 2000) found in position 3351 to 3748 of the genomic sequence shown in *Figure 11*. The B1 repetitive element is the mouse equivalent of the human Alu family of repeats. B1 repeats have the approximate size of 130 bp and are characterized by an A-rich tract at their 3´end (at position 3755 to 3831). They are often flanked by short direct repeats at their site of insertion in the genome (not seen in the murine CXCL11 sequence). Occasionally, repetitive elements are located in the 3´ UTR of mRNAs (King D et al. 1986). The presence of a B1 repetitive element in the mRNA of mouse genes is also known from other cDNAs (Zechner R et al. 1991).

Polymorphism

An alignment of the human CXCL11 cDNAs isolated from different sources showed sequence variations in the 3´ UTR in THP-1 cells. We confirmed these sequence deviations on the genomic sequence and defined a polymorphism in THP-1 cells. All variable positions in the 3′ UTR of CXCL11 were single nucleotides, 10 transitions and 1 transversion were detected and all are, silent. A further transition was detected in the 5′ UTR of the THP-1 cDNA type.

Whether these point mutations have an influence or not is unknown. It remains to be shown if other cells types show such a polymorphism or if these point mutations are characteristic only for THP-1. Already, their is some evidence for a polymorphism in the 3′UTR region of the mouse macrophage-like cell line RAW264.7 as well. Of note, a polymorphism is also reported in the 3′ UTR of murine CXCL10 (Hallensleben W et al. 2000).

In general, it is predicted that single nucleotide polymorphisms (SNPs) reflect past mutations that were mostly (but not exclusively) unique events. The phenomenon of SNPs becomes more and more important since many SNPs were found to be associated with human diseases. Furthermore, it is supposed that they provide a key to understand the human evolution (Stoneking M 2001).

Gene-family

The comparison of human and mouse CXCL11 could be extended to the two related chemokines CXCL10 and CXCL9 (Luster AD et al. 1985, Farber JM. 1990). Human CXCL9 (MIG) and CXCL10 (IP-10) and their murine homologues muCXCL9 (muMIG) and muCXCL10 (CRG-2 / muIP-10) have been identified several years before (Farber JM 1990), (Vanguri P and Farber JM. 1990) and are now well characterized.

A comparison of all three chemokines shows high similarities in the nucleotide and amino acid sequences. The amino acids encoded by the first exon constitute the signal peptide. These signal peptides are cleaved behind the first amino acid of the second exon (glycine in all three chemokines). The mature proteins of the related chemokines are of similar size: huCXCL11 is 73 amino acids in length, huCXCL10 is 77 amino acids and huCXCL9 is 103 amino acids in length. All three genes are composed of four exons with similar intron/exon structure (*Figure 8*). The high degree of relationship of these three proteins is further underlined by their expression pattern and their biological activity.

CXCL11, CXCL10 and CXCL9 are induced in a variety of cell types by IFN-γ and each of these chemokines is a ligand for CXCR3. CXCR3 is predominantly expressed on activated Th1 cells. For more details see Introduction, <u>chapter 2.5. Expression of CXCR3</u>. Thus, all three chemokines contribute to Th1-type immune responses by recruiting CXCR3 positive Th1 cells. The existence of multiple ligands for a single receptor is a common theme in the chemokine superfamily (Hughes A and Yeager M 1999).

A similar picture is observed in mice. The intron/exon organization of murine *Scyb11* is in line with our findings for human SCYB9-11 and murine *Scyb10* chemokines. For murine *Scyb9* this is also supposed but cannot be shown, since the genomic sequence is still not available in GenBank. The analogous murine receptor muCXCR3, which is 86 % identical to the human receptor, was cloned and shown to attract activated Th1 cells (Lu B et al. 1999). We could recently show that also in mice, all three chemokines stimulate this receptor with a hierarchy of potential similar to humans (Meyer M et al. submitted).

CXCL9, CXCL10 and CXCL11 form a distinct subgroup of chemokines showing similar expression pattern and function. A phylogenetic tree analysis of all human and murine CXC-chemokines available from GenBank showed that CXCL11, CXCL10 and CXCL9 share an individual branch on the evolutionary tree. See *Figure 10* for the human CXC chemokine dendrogram and *Figure 15* for the mouse CXC chemokine dendrogram.

Taken together, these data indicate a high degree of conservation for these CXC chemokine sequences concerning structure and function. Therefore, mouse models of human diseases are likely to yield relevant findings on the role of these chemokines in various human diseases.

Gene-arrangement

Human SCYB9, SCYB10 and SCYB11 are physically linked within a minicluster on human chromosome 4 and the syntenic mouse chromosome 5. The fibre-FISH experiments indicate that the three related genes in both human and mouse are similarly arranged in a cluster within a region of 29 kb on human chromosome 4q21 and of 32 kb on the orthologous mouse chromosome 5E3 (Erdel M et al. submitted). By combining our mapping results and the published data, additionally the alignment from centromere to telomere and the orientation in a head-to-tail manner of all three chemokine genes of the human 4q21 minicluster could be specified (O´Donovan N et al. 1999, Lee HH and Farber JM. 1996).

Nearly all chemokines are clustered: a main cluster and a separated mini-cluster are found for CC-chemokines on chromosome 17 and for CXC-chemokines on chromosome 4 in various species e.g. in human, mouse and cow (Modi WS et al. 1998). Gene clusters are also known for other immune relevant genes e.g. HLA-genes.

The explanations for these clustering are speculative. An obvious proposal for linkage of a set of genes is historical. This suggested that these genes evolved from a common ancestor by gene duplication. Another speculation is that some degree of coordinate regulation is achieved by clustering functionally linked genes together.

Our findings upon human and murine SCYB11 support the idea that the three genes CXCL9, CXCL10 and CXCL11 arose by gene duplication from a common precursor during mammalian evolution. However, if a common regulation of SCYB9, SCYB10 and SCYB11 exists, remains to be seen.

V. Summary

1. Summary in English

Chemokines are defined as small proteins, which regulate cell trafficking of various types of leukocytes. They can be subdivided into four groups due to their arrangement of the N-terminal cysteine(s): CC-chemokines have the first two cysteine residues adjacent, CXC-chemokines have an amino acid between these first two cysteines, CX_3C-chemokines have three variable amino acids in between, and the C-chemokines have only one cysteine residue at the N-terminus.

Among CXC chemokines, CXCL9 (alias MIG), CXCL10 (alias IP-10) and CXCL11 (alias βR1, H174, I-TAC, SCYB9B, IP-9) form a distinct branch on the evolutionary tree. They all lack the ELR-motif (glutamic acid-leucin-arginin) near the N-terminus and are ligands for the same receptor CXCR3, which is selectively expressed on activated Th1 cells. Furthermore, they have a similar expression pattern, as they are predominantly induced by interferon-γ and are produced by macrophages and numerous other cell types (Laich A et al. 1999, Cole KE et al. 1998, Tensen CP et al. 1999b).

In this work the genomic features of the CXC-chemokine CXCL11 (gene name SCYB11) was investigated. First, we isolated the cDNA of human CXCL11 from IFN-γ treated THP-1 cells. The cDNA encodes a 94 amino acid precursor protein, with a putative 21 amino acid signal peptide. By custom service, a genomic PAC library was screened and two clones carrying the SCYB11 gene were isolated. From one of these PAC clones, we subcloned the genomic sequence and about 3500 bp of the promoter region. SCYB11 expands over four exons and the exon/intron structure shows significant similarities to the two most related chemokine genes SCYB9 and SCYB10.

The promoter region contains various binding sites for regulatory elements, including four different IFN-responsive elements and one NF-κB site within 410 bp next to the start site. A functional promoter analysis was carried out, by cloning various huSCYB11 promoter elements into the pGL3 expression vector. The strongest induction was observed by IFN-γ followed by a good induction upon IFN-β and the combination TNF-α and IL-1. These findings are in line with mRNA expression data observed from various other cell types.

Since the cDNA of CXCL11 was published independently by different groups (Cole KE et al. 1998, Rani MRS et al. 1996, Jacobs KA et al. 1997), we could compare them and found some deviations. The cDNAs isolated from different cell types were found to use varying poly-adenylation signals which are tandemly arranged in the 3′ UTR region. Furthermore, an alignment of these cDNAs identified a polymorphism of CXCL11 in THP-1 cells. Twelve single nucleotide exchanges were found in the 3′ UTR region, but all are supposed to be silent.

The PAC clone was further used to map the SCYB11 gene to chromosome 4 position q21.2 and for fibre-FISH experiments. With this fine mapping, we could show that all three related chemokine genes SCYB9, SCYB10 and SCYB11 are on the same PAC clone and are arranged in a chromosomal minicluster of 29 kb.

The homologous murine sequence cDNA muCXCL11 was isolated from RAW264.7 cells treated with interferon-γ and LPS. The cDNA sequence of murine CXCL11 shares 63 % identity with its human counterpart, encoding for a 100 amino acid precursor protein with a putative signal peptide of 21 amino acids. Recently, we could show, that the synthetically prepared muCXCL11 protein binds to the murine CXCR3 receptor (homologue to human CXCR3) and induces an intracellular calcium influx (Meyer M et al. submitted). Like human CXCL11, the use of alternative polyadenylation signals was observed. The genomic sequence was determined with the Genome Walking strategy. The murine Scyb11 gene contains two repetitive elements: in intron 1 a 201 bp stretch of high cryptic simplicity and in the 3′ UTR region a B1 repetitive sequence followed by the typical A-rich trace was found. A comparison of human and murine Scyb11 showed a highly similar organization in four exons similar to the related murine Scyb10 sequence. (Gene sequence of Scyb9 is not available.) The murine Scyb11 promoter is known up to base -447. Within this region, several transcription regulatory elements are found by computer-assisted analysis. Of note, a 190 bp region of the murine Scyb11 promoter shows high similarity to the human SCYB11 promoter including important regulatory elements like the NF-κB and ISRE site and the TATA-box, which are conserved in their relative position and distance in the human and mouse SCYB11 promoter.

A genomic BAC clone containing murine Scyb11 was used for chromosomal mapping of the gene to mouse chromosome 5E3, which is orthologous to human 4q21.2 region. Furthermore, the BAC clone was used for fibre FISH experiments. Comparing the fibre-FISH data from man and mouse SCYB9-11 genes, shows similar arrangements in a cluster in orthologous chromosome locations.

These findings suggest that all three genes have evolved from a common ancestor by gene duplication and that this duplication occurred before the branching of the Rodent and Primate lineages.

2. Zusammenfassung in Deutsch

Chemokine, eine Unterfamilie der Cytokine, sind kleine sekretorische Proteine, die chemotaktisch auf Leukozyten wirken. Die Chemokin Familie wird anhand der Cystein-Anordnung in ihrer Aminosäure Sequenz in zwei Haupt und zwei Nebengruppen unterteilt: Die Hauptgruppen bilden die CC-Chemokine, bei denen die ersten beiden Cysteine direkt nebeneinander liegen und die CXC-Chemokine, bei denen diese beiden Cysteine durch eine variable Aminosäure getrennt sind. Die zwei Nebengruppen mit jeweils nur einem bekannten Vertreter bilden die CX_3C-Chemokine mit drei variablen Aminosäuren zwischen den ersten beiden Cysteinen und die C-Chemokine mit nur einem Cystein am N-Terminus.

Innerhalb der CXC-Chemokine bilden CXCL9 (alias MIG), CXCL10 (alias IP-10) und CXCL11 (alias βR1, H174, I-TAC, SCYB9B, IP-9) in struktureller und funktioneller Hinsicht eine Untergruppe. Allen drei Chemokinen fehlt das für alle anderen CXC-Chemokine typische ELR-Motiv. Weiters sind sie Liganden für denselben Rezeptor, CXCR3, und wirken chemotaktisch auf aktivierte Th 1 Zellen, während die meisten anderen CXC-Chemokine Neutrophile anlocken. Eine weitere Gemeinsamkeit ist das sehr ähnliche Expressionsmuster, der Hauptstimulus ist IFN-γ.

In der vorliegenden Arbeit wurden die genomischen Charakteristika des CXC-Chemokins CXCL11 (Genname SCYB11) untersucht. Dafür wurde die cDNA für humanes CXCL11 aus IFN-γ stimulierten THP-1 Zellen isoliert. Die cDNA kodiert ein 94 Aminosäuren Vorläufer-Protein mit einem 21 Aminosäure langen Signalpeptid am N-Terminus. Ausgehend von der cDNA wurde eine genomische PAC Bibliothek durchsucht, aus der zwei positive Klone isoliert werden konnten. Von einem der beiden Klone wurde die Gensequenz und rund 3500 bp der Promoterregion subkloniert. Das Gen von SCYB11 erstreckt sich über vier Exons und ist in der

Exon/Intron Aufteilung den beiden verwandten Genen SCYB9 und SCYB10 sehr ähnlich.

Im weiteren wurde die Promoterregion analysiert und vielfältige Bindungsstellen für regulatorische Elemente entdeckt. Insbesondere in der dem Transkriptionsstart nächstgelegenen Region wurden wichtige Bindungsstellen, darunter vier verschiedene IFN-regulatorische Elemente und eine NF-κB Bindungsstelle gefunden. Die Funktion des Promoters ist durch Klonierung in den pGL3 Expressionsvektor bestätigt worden. Unter den zahlreichen Stimuli, die ausgetestet wurden, ist IFN-γ der stärkste Induktor. Ebenso erwiesen sich IFN-β und die Kombination von IL-1β und TNF-α als gute Stimulanzien. Die Resultate der funktionellen Promoteranalyse stimmen mit bereits bekannten mRNA Expressions- Daten weitgehend überein (Laich A et al. 1999, Rani MRS et al. 1996, Cole KE et al. 1998).

Die CXCL11 cDNA wurde von mehren Arbeitsgruppen unabhängig isoliert und publiziert (Cole KE et al. 1998, Rani MRS et al. 1996, Jacobs KA et al. 1997). Bei einem Vergleich fallen zwei Abweichungen auf: Die cDNAs, die aus verschiedenen Zelltypen isoliert wurden, haben verschieden lange 3′ UTR. Dieser Unterschied kommt durch die Nutzung verschiedener Polyadenylierungs-Stellen, die in einer Tandem-Anordnung in der 3′ UTR Region liegen, zustande. Außerdem konnte durch Aufstapelung verschiedener cDNA Sequenzen ein Polymorphismus in THP-1 Zellen entdeckt werden. Die SCYB11 cDNA, isoliert aus THP-1 Zellen, enthält zwölf Punktmutationen, die keinen Einfluss auf den Leserahmen haben.

Mit FISH Experimenten, durchgeführt von Martin Erdel (Institut für Medizinische Biologie an der Universität Innsbruck) konnte SCYB11 am humanen Chromosom 4q21.2 lokalisiert werden. Diesem Genlokus wurde in früheren Arbeiten SCYB9 und SCYB10 zugeordnet. Mit Faser-FISH, konnte die genaue Anordnung der drei verwandten Chemokin Gene SCYB9, SCYB10 and SCYB11 in enger Nachbarschaft von 29 kb nachgewiesen werden (Erdel M et al. submitted).

Die homologe Maus Sequenz muCXCL11 cDNA wurde aus IFN-γ stimulierten RAW264.7 Zellen isoliert. Die murine cDNA Sequenz stimmt zu 63 % mit der humanen cDNA überein. Die cDNA kodiert ein 100 Aminosäuren langes Vorläufer-Peptid, mit einem 21 Aminosäure langen Signalpeptid. Für das reife, 79 Aminosäuren lange muCXCL11 Protein (synthetisch hergestellt) konnte kürzlich die chemotaktische Anlockung von Zellen, die den murinen CXCR3 Rezeptor exprimieren, nachgewiesen werden (Meyer M et al. submitted).

Die genomische Sequenz wurde mit der "Genome Walking" Technik isoliert. Beim Maus Gen fallen zwei repetitive Elemente auf: zum einen im Intron 1 eine 201 bp lange Abfolge von TTTC, CTTC, TTCC und TC, zum anderen in der 3′ UTR Region ein B1 Element mit einer daran anschließenden A-reichen Region.

Ein Vergleich der Intron/Exon Struktur von humanem und murinem SCYB11 zeigt eine sehr ähnliche Aufteilung. Ebenso ist die Intron/Exon Aufteilung des verwandten murinen Chemokines *Scyb10* sehr ähnlich.

Der Promoter von Maus *Scyb11* wurde bis Base -447 isoliert. Innerhalb dieser Region konnten mehrere Bindungsstellen für regulatorische Elemente mit Computerunterstützter Analyse nachgewiesen werden. Besonders interessant ist, dass zwischen murinem und humanem Promoter eine Region von 190 bp starke Ähnlichkeit aufweist. Innerhalb dieser Region stimmen wichtige transkriptions-regulatorische Elemente wie eine NF-κB Stelle, die ISRE Stelle und die TATA-box in ihrer Position zueinander und zum Transkriptionsstart überein.

Ein genomischer BAC Klon, auf dem sich die Sequenz von *Scyb11* befindet, wurde für die chromosomale Lokalisation verwendet. Das murine *Scyb11* wurde Chromosom 5E3 zugeordnet, einer orthologen Genregion zum humanen 4q21.2. Faser-FISH Experimente, die ebenfalls mit diesem BAC Klon durchgeführt wurden, zeigen, dass die drei verwandten murinen Chemokine *Scyb9*, *Scyb10* und *Scyb11* in der gleichen Anordnung wie beim Menschen, in einem engen Bereich von 32 kb liegen.

Diese Ergebnisse führen zu der Schlussfolgerung, dass die drei verwandten Chemokine, die in ihrer Exon/Intron Aufteilung, in ihrer Expression und Funktion so große Ähnlichkeit aufweisen, durch Genduplikation entstanden sind. Weiters ist zu vermuten, dass sich diese Duplikation zu einem Zeitpunkt in der Evolution ereignete, als sich die Nagetiere und die Primaten Linie noch nicht getrennt hatten.

VI. References

Ahuja SK, Murphy PM. Molecular piracy of mammalian interleukin-8 receptor type B by herpesvirus saimiri. J Biol Chem (1993) 268:20691- 20694

Alberts B, Bray D, Lewis J, Raff M, Roberts K, Watson JD. Molecular Biology of the Cell. Third Edition; New York: Garland Publishing Inc. (1994)

Baggiolini M, Walz A, Kunkel SL. Neutrophil-activation peptide-1/interleukin 5, a novel cytokine that activates neutrophils. J Clin Invest. (1989) 84: 1045-1049

Baggiolini M. Chemokines and leukocyte traffic. Nature (1998) 392: 565-568

Baggiolini M, Dewald B, Moser B. Interleukin-8 related chemotactic cytokines-CXC and CC chemokines. Adv Immunol (1994) 55: 97-179

Baggiolini M, Dewald B, Moser B. Human chemokines : an update. Annu Rev Immunol (1997) 15: 675-705

Baggiolini M, Moser B. Blocking chemokine receptors. J Exp Med (1997) 186(8): 1189-1191

Birnstiel ML, Busslinger M, Strub K. Transcription termination and 3´processing: the end is in site! Cell (1985) 41: 349-359

Bleul CC, Farzan M, Choe H, Paroli C, Clark-Lewis I, Sodroski J, Springer TA. The lymphocyte chemoattractant SDF-1 is a ligand for LESTR/fusin and blocks HIV-1 entry. (1996) Nature 382: 829-833

Bonecchi R, Bianchi G, Bordignon PP, D´Ambrosio D, Lang R, Borsatti A, Sozzani S, Allavena P, Gray PA, Mantovani A, Sinigaglia F. Differential expression of chemokine receptors and chemotactic responsiveness of type 1 T helper cells (Th1´s) and Th2´s. J Exp Med (1998) 187(1): 129-134

Böhm SK, Grady EF, Bunnett NW. Regulatory mechanisms that modulate signalling by G-protein-coupled receptors. Biochem J (1997) 322: 1-18

Butcher EC, Picker LJ. Lymphocyte homing and homeostasis. Science (1996) 272: 60-66

Chen CYA and SHYU AB. AU-rich elements: characterization and importance in mRNA degradation. Trends Biochem Sci (1995) 20: 465-470

Chomczynski P, Sacci N. Single-step method of RNA isolation by acid guanidinium thiocyanate-phenol-chloroform extraction. Anal Biochem (1987) 162: 156-159

Clark-Lewis I, Dewald B, Geiser T, Moser B, Baggiolini M. J Biol. Chem (1991) 266:18989-18994

Clark-Lewis I, Schumacher C, Baggiolini M, Moser B. Structure-acitivity relationships of interleukin-8 determined using chemically synthesized analogs. Critical role of NH_2-terminal residues and evidence for uncoupling of neutrophil chemotaxis, exocytosis, and receptor binding activities. J Biol Chem (1991) 266: 23128-23134

Clark-Lewis I, Dewald B, Geiser T, Moser B, Baggiolini M. Platelet factor 4 binds to interleukin 8 receptors and activates neutrophils when its N terminus is modified with Glu-Leu-Arg. Proc Natl Acad Sci USA (1993) 90: 3574-3577

Clark-Lewis I, Dewald B, Loetscher M, Moser B, Baggiolini M. Structural requirements for interleukin-8 function identified by design of analogs and CXC chemokine hybrids. J Biol Chem (1994) 269(23): 16075-16081

Cole KE, Strick CA, Paradis TJ, Ogborne KT, Loetscher M, Gladue RP, Lin W, Boyd JG, Moser B, Wood DE, Sahagan BG, Neote K. Interferon-inducible T cell alpha chemoattractant (I-TAC):

a novel non-ELR CXC chemokine with potent activity on activated T cells through selective high affinity binding to CXCR3. J Exp Med (1998) 187: 2009-2021

Crump MP, Gong JH, Loetscher P, Rajarathnam K, Amara A, Arenzana-Seisdedos F, Virelizier JL, Baggiolini M, Sykes BD, Clark-Lewis I. Solution structure and basis for functional activity of stromal cell-derived factor-1; dissociation of CXCR4 activation from binding and inhibition of HIV-1. EMBO J (1997) 23(16): 6996-7007

Devreotes PN, Zigmond SH. Chemotaxis in eukaryotic cells: a focus on leukocytes and Dictyostelium. Annu Rev Cell Biol (1988) 4: 649-686

Ebnet K, Simon MM, Shaw S. Regulation of chemokine gene expression in human endothelial cells by proinflammatory cytokines and Borrelia burgdorferi. Ann N Y Acad Sci (1996) 797: 107-117

Edwalds-Gilbert G, Veraldi KL, Milcarek C. Alternative poly(A) site selection in complex transcription units: means to an end? Nucleic Acid Res (1997) 25(13): 2547-2561

Erdel M, Laich A, Utermann G, Werner ER, Werner-Felmayer G. The human gene encoding SCYB9B, a putative novel CXC chemokine, maps to human chromosome 4q21 like the closely related genes for MIG (SCYB9) and INP 10 (SCYB10). Cytogenet Cell Genet (1998) 81: 271-272

Erdel M, Theurl M, Meyer M, Duba HC, Utermann G, Werner-Felmayer G. High-resolution mapping of the human 4q21 and the murine 5E3 SCYB chemokine cluster by fiber-FISH (2001) submitted

Farber JM. A macrophage mRNA selectively induced by γ-interferon encodes a member of the platelet factor 4 family of cytokines. Proc Natl Acad Sci (1990) 87: 5238-5242

Farber JM. A collection of mRNA species that are inducible in the RAW 264.7 mouse macrophage cell line by gamma interferon and other agents. Mol Cell Biol (1992) 12: 1535-1545

Farber JM. HuMIG: a new member of the chemokine family of cytokines. Biochem Biophys Res Comm (1993) 192: 223-230

Feniger-Barish R, Belkin D, Zaslaver A, Gal S, Dori M, Ran M, Ben-Baruch A. GCP-2-induced internalization of IL-8 receptors: hierarchical relationships between GCP-2 and other ELR(+) - CXC chemokines and mechanisms regulating CXCR2 internalization and recycling. Blood (2000) 95(5): 1551-1559

Foxman EF, Campbell JJ, Butcher EC. Multistep navigation and the combinatorial control of leukocyte chemotaxis. J Cell Biol (1997) 139(5): 1349-1360

Gale LM, McColl SR. Chemokines: extracellular messengers for all occasions? BioEssays (1999) 21: 17-28

Gao JL, Murphy PM. Human cytomegalovirus open reading frame US28 encodes a functional beta chemokine receptor. J Biol Chem (1994) 269: 28539-28542

Edwalds-Gilbert G, Veraldi KL, Milcarek C. Alternative poly(A) site selection in complex transcription units: means to an end? Nucleic Acids Res (1997) 25(13): 2547-2561

Gong W, Howard OM, Turpin JA, Grimm MC, Ueda H, Gray PW, Raport CJ, Oppenheim JJ, Wang JM. Monocyte chemotactic protein-2 activates CCR5 and blocks CD4/CCR5-mediated HIV-1 entry/replication. J Biol Chem (1998) 273(8): 4289-4292

Hallensleben W, Biro L, Sauder C, Hausmann J, Asensio V, Campbell IL, Staeheli P. A polymorphism in the mouse Crg-2 / IP-10 gene complicates chemokine gene expression analysis using a commercial ribonuclease protection assay. J Immunol Meth (2000) 234: 149-151

von Heijne G. Patterns of amino acids near signal-sequence cleavage sites. Eur J Biochem (1983) 133: 17-21

Henikoff S. Unidirectional digestion with exonuclease III in DNA sequence analysis. Meth Enzymol (1987) 155: 156-165

Hensbergen PJ, van der Raaij-Helmer EMH, Dijkman R, van der Schors RC, Werner-Felmayer G, Boorsma DM, Scheper RJ, Willemze R, Tensen C. Processing of natural and recombinant CXCR3 targeting chemokines and implications for biological activity; in prep.

Horuk R. Chemokine receptors and HIV-1: the fusion of the major research fields. Immunol Today. (1999) 20(2): 89-94

Hughes AL, Yeager M. Coevolution of the mammalian chemokines and their receptors. Immunogenetics. (1999) 49: 115-125

Ioannou PA, Amemiya CT, Garnes J, Kroisel PM, Shizuya H, Chen C, Batzer MA, deJong PJ. A new bacteriophage P1-derived vector for the propagation of large human DNA fragments Nat Genet (1994) 6:84-89

Jacobs KA, Collins-Racie LA, Colbert M, Duckett M, Golden-Fleet M, Kelleher K, Kriz R, La Vallie ER, Merberg D, Spaulding V, Stover J, Williamson MJ, McCoy JM. A genetic selection of isolation cDNAs encoding secreted proteins. Gene (1997) 198: 289-296

Kanegane C, Sgadari C, Kanegane H, Teruya-Feldstein J, Yao L, Gupta G, Farber JM, Liao F, Liu L, Tosato G. Contribution of the CXC chemokines IP-10 and MIG to the antitumoral effects of IL-12. J Leukoc Biol (1998) 64(3): 384-392

Kim UJ, Birren BW, Slepak T, Mancino V, Boysen C, Kang HL, Simon MI, Shizuya H. Construction and characterization of a human bacterial artificial chromosome library. Genomics (1996) 34: 213-218

King D, Snider LD, Lingrel JB. Polymorphism in an androgen-regulated mouse gene is the result of the insertion of a B1 repetitive element into the transcription unit. Mol Cell Biol (1986) 6: 209-217

Kozak M. Point mutations define a sequence flanking the AUG initiator codon that modulates translation by eukaryotic ribosomes. Cell (1986) 44: 283-292

Laich A, Meyer M, Werner ER, Werner-Felmayer G. Structure and expression of the human small cytokine B subfamily member 11 (SCYB11/formerly SCYB9B, alias I-TAC) gene cloned from IFN-γ-treated human monocytes (THP-1). J Interferon Cytokine Res (1999) 19: 505-513

Lee HH, Farber JM. Localization of the gene for the human MIG cytokine on chromosome 4q21 adjacent to INP10 reveals a chemokine "minicluster". Cytogenet Cell Genet (1996) 74: 255-258

Liao F, Rabin RL, Yannelli JR, Koniaris LG, Vanguri P, Farber JM. Human Mig chemokine: biochemical and functional characterization. J Exp Med (1995) 182: 1301-1314

Loetscher ML, Gerber B, Loetscher P, Jones SA, Piali L, Clark-Lewis IC, Baggiolini M, Moser B. Chemokine receptor specific for IP-10 and MIG: structure, function and expression in activated T lymphocytes. J Exp Med (1996) 184: 963-969

Loetscher P, Pellegrion A, Gong JH, Mattioli I, Loetscher M, Bardi G, Baggiolini M, Clark-Lewis I. The ligands of CXC chemokines receptor 3, I-TAC, MIG and IP-10, are natural antagonists for CCR3. J Biol Chem. in press

Lu B, Humbles A, Bota D, Gerard C, Moser B, Soler D; Luster AD; Gerard N. Structure and function of the murine chemokine receptor CXCR3. Eur J Immunol (1999) 29: 3804-3812

Luster AD, Unkeless JC, Ravetch JV. γ-Interferon transcriptionally regulates an early-response gene containing homology to platelet proteins. Nature (1985) 315:672-676

Luster AD, Ravetch JV. Genomic characterization of a gamma-interferon-inducible gene (IP-10) and identification of an interferon-inducible hypersensitive site. Mol Cell Biol (1987) 7(10): 3723-3731

Mach F, Sauty A, Iarossi AS, Sukhova GK, Neote K, Libby P, Luster AD. Differential expression of three T lymphocyte-activating CXC chemokines by human atheroma-associated cells. J Clin Invest (1999) 104(8): 1041-1050

Majumder S, Zhou LZH, Chaturvedi P, Babcock G, Aras S, Ransohoff RM. Regulation of human IP-10 gene expression in astrocytoma cells by inflammatory cytokines. J Neuroscience Res (1998) 54: 169-180

Mellado M, Rodriguez-Frade JM, Vila-Coro AJ, de Ana AM, Martinez-AC. Chemokine control of HIV-1 infection. Nature (1999) 400: 723-724

Meyer M, Erdel M, Duba HC, Werner ER, Werner-Felmayer G. Cloning, genomic sequence, and chromosome mapping of *SCYB11*, the murine homologue of SCYB11 (alias β-R1/H174/SCYB9B/I-TAC/IP-9/CXCL11). Cytogenet Cell Genet (2000) 88: 278-282

Meyer M, Hensbergen PJ, van der Raaij-Helmer EMH, Brandacher G, Margreiter R, Heufler C, Koch F, Narumi S, Werner ER, Colvin R, Luster AD, Tensen CP, Werner-Felmayer G. Cross reactivity of three T-cell attracting murine chemokines stimulating the CXC chemokine receptor CXCR3 and their induction in cultured cells and during allograft rejection. (2001) submitted

Modi WS, Amarante MRV, Hanson M, Womack JE, Chidambaram A. Assignment of the mouse and cow CXC chemokine genes. Cytogenet Cell Genet (1998) 81: 213-216

Modi WS, Chen ZQ. Localization of the human CXC chemokine subfamily on the long arm of chromosome 4 using radiation hybrids (1998) 47: 136-139

Nomiyama H, Fukuda S, Masayoshi I, Tanase S, Miura R, Yoshie O. Organization of the chemokine gene cluster of human chromosome 17q11.2 containing the genes for CC chemokines MPIF-1, HCC-2, HCC-1, LEC, and RANTES. J Interf Cytok Res (1999) 19: 227-234

O'Donovan N, Galvin M, Morgan JG. Physical mapping of the CXC chemokine locus on human chromosome 4. Cytogent Cell Genet (1999) 84: 39-42

Ogg SL, Komaragiri MVS, Mather IH. Structural organization and mammary-specific expression of the butyrophilin gene. Mamm Genom (1996) 7: 900-905

Ohmori Y, Hamilton TA. Cooperative interaction between interferon (IFN) stimulus response element and κB sequence motifs controls IFN-γ and lipopolysaccharide-stimulated transcription from the murine IP-10 promoter. J Biol Chem (1993) 268(9): 6677-6688

Ohmori Y, Schreiber RD, Hamilton TA. Synergy between interferon-γ and tumor necrosis factor-α in transcriptional activation is mediated by cooperation between signal transducer and activator of transcription 1 and nuclear factor κB. J Biol Chem (1997) 272(23): 14899-14907

Parra I, Windle B. High resolution visual mapping of stretched DNA by fluorescent hybridization. Nature Genetics (1993) 5: 17-21

Piali L, Weber C, LaRosa G, Mackay CR, Springer TA, Clark-Lewis I, Moser B. The chemokine receptor CXCR3 mediates rapid and shear-resistant adhesion-induction of effector T lymphocytes by the chemokines IP-10 and MIG. Eur J Immunol (1998) 28(3): 961-972

Qin S, Rooman JB, Myers P, Kassam N, Weinblatt M, Loetscher M, Koch AE, Moser B, Mackay CR. The chemokine receptors CXCR3 and CCR5 mark subsets of T cells associated with certain inflammatory reactions. J Clin Invest (1998) 101(4): 746-754

Rani MRS, Foster GR, Leung S, Leaman D, Stark GR, Ransohoff RM. Characterization of β-R1, a gene that is selectively induced by interferon β (IFN-β) compared with IFN-alpha. J Biol Chem (1996) 271: 22878-22884

Sallusto F, Kremmer E, Palermo B, Hoy A, Ponath P, Qin S, Förster R, Lipp M, Lanzavecchia A. Switch in chemokine receptor expression upon TCR stimulation reveals novel homing potential for recently activated T cells. Eur J Immunol (1999) 29: 2037-2045

Sallusto F, Mackay CR, Lanzavecchia A. The role of chemokine receptors in primary, effector, and memory immune responses. Annu Rev Immunol (2000) 18: 593-620

Sarris AH, Broxmyer HE, Wirthmuller U, Karasavvas N, Cooper S, Lu L, Krueger J, Ravetch JV. Human interferon inducible protein 10: expression and purification of recombinant protein demonstrate inhibition of early human hematopoietic progenitors. J Exp Med (1993) 178: 1127-1132

Sauty A, Wagner L, Mach F, Yang OO, Neote K, Libby P, Luster AD. IP-10, MIG and I-TAC are highly expressed by IFN-γ-activated human endothelial cells, but only I-TAC strongly induces CXCR3 internalization. Abstractbook of Keystone Symposia (Chemokines and Chemokines Receptor) (1999) 38

Sen GC, Lengyel P. The interferon system: a bird eye view of its biochemistry. J Biol Chem (1992) 267(8): 5017-5020

Seyffert W, Gasser HG, Hess O, Jäckle H, Fischbach KF. Lehrbuch der Genetik; First Edition (1998) Stuttgart Gustav Fischer Verlag

Sgadari C, Farber JM, Angiolillio AL, Liao F, Teryua-Feldstein J, Burd PR, Yao L, Gupta G, Kanegane C, TosatoG. Mig, the monokine induced by interferon-gamma, promotes tumor necrosis in vivo. Blood (1997) 89(8): 2635-2643

Shirozu M, Nakano T, Inazawa J, Tashiro K, Tada H, Shinohara T, Honjo T. Structure and chromosomal localization of the human stromal cell-derived factor 1 (SDF1) gene. Genomics (1995) 28: 495-500

Springer TA. Traffic signals for lymphocytes recirculation and leukocyte emigration: the multistep paradigm. Cell (1994) 76: 301-314

Stryer L. Biochemie, fourth edition. Spectrum Akademischer Verlag Heidelberg, Berin, Oxford (1996)

Stoneking M. Single nucleotide polymorphism: from the evolutionary past... Nature (2001) 409: 824-822

Strieter RM, Polverini PJ, Kunkel SL, Arenberg DA, Burdick MD, Kasper J, Dzuiba J, VanDamme J, Walz A, Marriott D, Chan SY, Roczniak S, Shanafelt AB. The functional role of the ELR motif in CXC chemokines-mediated angiogenesis. J Biol Chem (1995) 270: 27348-27357

Tanaka N, Kawakami T, Taniguchi T. Recognition DNA sequences of interferon regulatory factor 1 (IRF-1) and IRF-2, regulators of cell growth and the interferon system. Mol Cell Biol (1993) 13(8): 4513-4538

Tautz D, Renz M. Simple sequences are ubiquitous repetitive components of eukaryotic genomes. Nucleic Acid Res (1984) 12: 4127-4139

Tautz D, Schlötterer C. Simple sequences. Curr Biol (1994) 4: 832-837

Tensen CP, Flier J, van der Raaij-Helmer EMH, Sampat-Sardjoepersad S, van der Schors RC, Leurs R, Scheper RJ, Boorsma DM, Willemze R. Human IP-9: a kertinocyte-derived high affinity CXC-chemokine ligand for the IP-10/MIG receptor (CXCR3). J Invest Dermatol (1999a) 112(5): 716-722

Tensen CP, Flier J, Rampersad SS, Sampat-Sardjoepersad S, Scheper RJ, Boorsma DM, Willemze R. Genomic organization, sequence and transcriptional regulation of the human CXCL11 gene. Biochim Biophys Acta (1999b) 1446: 167-172

Tunnacliffe A, Majumdar S, Yan B, Poncz M. Genes for β-thromboglobulin and platelet factor 4 are closely linked and form part of a cluster of related genes on chromosome 4. Blood (1992) 79: 2896-2900

Vanguri P, Farber JM. Identification of CRG-2, an interferon-inducible mRNA predicted to encode a murine monokine. J Biol Chem (1990) 265(5): 15049-15057

Werner ER, Werner-Felmayer G, Mayer G. Tetrahydobiopterin, cytokines, and nitric oxide synthesis. Proc Soc Exp Biol Med (1998) 219: 171-182

Widney DP, Xia YR, Lusis AJ, Smith JB. The murine chemokine CXCL11 (IFN-inducible T cell α chemoattractant) is an IFN-γ- and lipopolysaccaride-inducible glucocorticoid-attenuated response gene expressed in lung and other tissues during endotoxemia. J Immunol (2000) 164: 6322-6331

Wong P, Severns CW, Guyer NB, Wright TM. A unique palindromic element mediates gamma interferon induction of mig gene expression. Mol Cell Biol (1994) 14(2): 914-992

Wright TM, Farber JM. 5′ Regulatory region of a novel cytokine gene mediates selective activation by interferon γ. J Exp Med (1991) 173: 417-422

Zechner R, Newman TC, Steiner E, Breslow JL. The structure of the mouse lipoprotein lipase gene: a B1 repetitive element is inserted into the 3′ untranslated region of the mRNA. Genomics (1991) 11: 62-76

Zlotnik A, Yoshie O. Chemokines: a new classification system and their role in immunity. Immunity (2000) 12: 121-127

VII. Appendix

1. List of regulatory elements found in the promoter region

transcription factor	matrix	short description

AP-1
AP-1_C
AP-1Q2

enhancer
    down modulated by glucocorticoids through direct interaction with glucocorticoid receptor;

c-REL
CREL_01

enhancer
    acts as potent activator as homodimer or heterodimer with RelA
has an overlapping DNA binding specificity with NF–κB

GATA-1
GATA1_02
GATA1_03
GATA1_04

negative regulator
    in association with SP1 or CCAACC binding proteins; Zinc-finger

GR-alpha
GRE_C

activator or repressor
    in response to glucocorticoid hormones; cooperation with transcription factors

HSF1
(heat shock transcription factor 1)
HSF1_01

activator
    mediating response to heat, stress and heavy metals;

IRF-1 = ISGF-2
IRF-1_01

activator
    positive regulator of interferon-beta and interferon inducible genes;
same DNA binding specificity as IRF-2;

IRF-2	*IRF-2_01*	<u>negative regulator</u> of interferon-beta expression, same DNA binding specificity as IRF-1
ISGF-3	*ISRE_01*	<u>activator</u> / multimeric complex rapid interferon response factor;
NF-_B (homologue EBP-1)	*NF-_B50_01* *NF_B65_01* *NF_B_01* *NF_B_C* *NF_B_Q6*	<u>activator</u> key regulator of genes involved in responses to infection, inflammation, stress; induced by many agents like TNF-α and dsRNA constituted either by a p50 homodimer, a p50/p65 heterodimer or heterotetramer
NF-IL6 (synonym C/EBP beta CeBP delta)	*CEBPB_01* *CEBPB_02*	<u>activator</u> induced by LPS or inflammatory cytokines; involved in acute phase reaction, inflammation and hematopoiesis; may heterodimerize with either c–Fos or c–Jun
OCT-1	*OCT1_02* *OCT1_07* *OCT1_C* *OCT1_06* *OCT1_05*	<u>transcription activator</u> in the Pol II and Pol III system cooperative effects with SP-1 and PR;
Sp-1	*SP1_Q6* *SP1_01*	<u>activator</u> highly specific cooperation with NF-κB; effect of SP-1 sites depends on distance to TATA–Box; multimerisation leads to super activation

GAS   *STAT1_01*   <u>activator</u>
(STAT 1 homodimer)   *STAT_01*   signal to induction of interferon-stimulated gene
                                       expression;
                                       induced by IFN-α, IFN-γ, and growth factors

STAT 2   *STAT_01*   <u>transcription activator</u>
                                               kinase which response to IFN-α but not IFN–γ;
                                       enhances formation of ISGF3 complex

STAT 3   *STAT3_01*   <u>transcription activator</u>
                                               activated by EGF and IL-6, not by IFN–γ, by
                                       tyrosine phosphorylation

2. Solutions

Ampicillin-Stock Solution 50x

250 mg ampicillin

9 ml aqua dest

1 drop of NaOH to get ampicillin solved

bring volume to 10 ml

store to -20 °C

Choramphenicol-Stock Solution 100x

25 mg chloramphenicol

1 ml ethanol absolute

store at -20 °C

CTAB / Hexadecyltrimethly Ammonium Bromide

0,5 g Hexadecyltrimethly Ammonium Bromide

9 ml aqua dest.

dissolve at 37 °C

add 1ml sodium chloride 5 M

Denaturation Solution

20 g sodium hydroxide

87.7 g sodium chloride

Denhardt 100x

10 g Ficoll 400

10 g polyvinylpyrrolidone

10 g BSA

bring volume to 500 ml with aqua dest.

dNTP Mixture, 10 mM

    2 µl 100 mM stock solution of dATP

    2 µl 100 mM stock solution of dCTP

    2 µl 100 mM stock solution of dGTP

    2 µl 100 mM stock solution of dTTP

Ethidium Bromide

    dissolve 10 mg/ml ethidium bromide in aqua dest.

    store at 4 °C

EDTA 0.5 M, pH 8

    186.1 g EDTA (Tritriplex III)

    dissolve in aqua dest.

    adjust pH to 8.0

    bring volume to 1 l with aqua dest.

Fish Sperm DNA

    dissolve 10 mg/ml deoxyribonucleic acid (from salmon testes) in aqua dest

    denaturation: place in 95 °C water bath for 5 min and then immediately on ice

Formamide deionised

    200 ml formamide

    10 g 501-x8 Resin (mixed bed resin)

    mix for 1 hour at room temperature

    filter through folded filter

Hybridisation Solution for Northern blot

    5 g dextrane sulphate

    70 mg sodium pyrophosphate

    dissolve in 30 ml at 37 °C

7.5 ml 20x SSC

5 ml 100x Denhardt

250 µl 20 % SDS

500 µl fish DNA

bring volume to 50 ml with aqua dest.

let mixture rest for several hours to allow proper dissolution

Hybridisation Solution for Southern blot

25 ml formamide deionised

12.5 ml SSPE 20x

2.5 ml Denhardt 100x

1.25 ml SDS 20 %

500 µl fish DNA

bring volume to 50 ml with aqua dest

IPTG 0.4 M

9.5 g isopropyl-1-thio-D-galactoside

dissolve in aqua dest.

bring volume to 100 ml

filter sterilize

Kanamycin-Stock Solution 100x

250 mg kanamycin monosulphate

dissolve in aqua dest.

bring volume to 10 ml

filter sterilize

store at -20 °C

KAc 5 M, pH 5.1

15 ml aqua dest.

15 ml acetic acid 100 %

add 7.5 g potassium hydroxide

adjust pH to 5.1

bring volume to 50 ml

Klenow-Fragment Buffer 10x

500 mM Tris, pH 8.0

50 mM $MgCl_2$

100 mM 2-mercaptoethanol

120 µM dATP

120 µM dGTP

120 µM dTTP

bring volume to 1 ml with aqua dest

store at -20 °C

LB-broth containing less sodium chloride

10 g tryptone peptone

5 g yeast extract

5 g sodium chloride

bring volume to 1 l with aqua dest

adjust pH to 7.4

autoclave

Loading Buffer

50 % glycerol

1 mM EDTA pH 8.5

0.5 % bromphenol blue

0.4 % xylene cyanol

autoclave

store at -20 °C

Ligase Mix

480 µl H_2O

60 µl ligase buffer

60 µl PEG 50 %

1.5 µl ligase

Lysozyme solution

dissolve 50 mg lysozyme in 1 ml aqua dest

make solution fresh before use

MOPS 10x

10.4 g MOPS

1.64 g sodium acetate

0,93 g EDTA

dissolve in aqua dest.

adjust pH to 7.0

bring volume to 250 ml with aqua dest.

filter sterilize

NaOH / SDS Solution

5 ml NaOH 2 M

2.5 ml SDS 20 %

bring volume to 50 ml

Neutralization Solution

60.5 g Tris

87.7 g sodium chloride

dissolve in aqua dest.

adjust pH to 7.4

bring volume to 1 l

PBS

9.55 g buffer substance Dulbecco´s powder

dissolve in aqua dest

bring volume to 1 l

filter sterilize

RNA loading mix (for 13 RNA samples)

45 µl formaldehyde

130 ml deionised formamide

13 µl MOPS 10x

13 µl sterile aqua dest

make mixture fresh before use

a 15 ml of this mixture are add to each RNA sample

RNase A Solution

100 mg RNase A

dissolve in 10 ml 10 mM Tris pH 7.4 and 15 mM NaCl

cook 10 min at 100 °C

let slowly cool to room temperature

S1 Stop Solution

3.6 g Tris (no HCl)

10 ml EDTA 0.5 M pH 8.0

bring volume to 100 ml

SDS 20 %

20 g sodium dodecyl sulphate

dissolve in aqua dest.

bring volume to 100 ml with aqua dest.

Sodium Acetate 3 M; pH 5.5

20.4 g sodium acetate

dissolve in aqua dest

bring volume to 50 ml

SSC 20x

> sodium chloride 3 M
>
> tri-sodium citrate dihydrate 0.2 M
>
> adjust pH to 7.0

SSPE 20x

> 210 g sodium chloride
>
> 27.6 g di-sodium hydrogen phosphate dodecalydrate
>
> 40 ml EDTA 0.5 M
>
> adjust pH to 7.4
>
> bring volume to 1 l

STET Buffer

> 4 g sucrose
>
> 1.5 ml Triton X-100
>
> 5 ml EDTA 0.5 M, pH 8.0
>
> 2.5 ml Tris 1 M, pH 8.0

TB-Medium (part I)

> 12 g tryptone peptone
>
> 24 g yeast extract
>
> 4.6 ml glycerol 87 %
>
> bring volume to 1 l
>
> autoclave

TB-Medium (part II)

> 2,3 g potassium dihydrogen phosphate
>
> 16,4 g di-potassium hydrogen phosphate
>
> bring volume to 100 ml
>
> autoclave

TB-Medium complete

> part I and II of the TB-medium have to be autoclaved
> separately to avoid precipitation
> mix part I and part II in a ratio of 9:1

TBE Buffer 10x

> 108 g Tris
> 55 g boric acid
> 40 ml 0.5M EDTA, pH 8.0
> bring volume to 1 l with aqua dest

TBE Buffer 1x supplemented with Ethidiumbromide

> 100 ml 10x TBE
> 900 ml aqua dest
> 70 µl 10 mg/ml ethidiumbromide

TE Buffer, pH 8.0

> 10 mM Tris
> 1 M EDTA
> adjust pH to 8.0
> filter sterilize

Tetracycline Stock Solution 100x

> 12.5 mg/ml tetracycline hydrochloride
> dissolve in ethanol abs./aqua dest 50 % V/V
> filter sterilize
> store at -20 °C

Trituration Buffer

> 100 mM calcium chloride
> 70 mM magnesium chloride
> 40 mM sodium acetate pH 5.5

bring volume to 100 ml

filter sterilize

prepare buffer always fresh

Tris/EDTA/Glucose Solution

12.5 ml Tris 1 M pH 8.0

5 ml EDTA 0.5 M pH 8.0

0.5g glucose

dissolve in 50 ml aqua dest.

filter sterilize

Tris-HCl 1 M, pH 8.5

12.1 g Tris

dissolve in aqua dest.

adjust pH to 8.5

with HCl

X-Gal

dissolve 20 mg/ml 5-bromo-4-chloro-3-indolyl-beta-D-

galactoside in

sterile dimethlyformamide

store in dark glass at 4 °C

3. Chemicals

Albumin bovine Fraction V / BSA   Serva Electrophoresis, Heidelberg, Germany
pH 7.0

Ammonium acetate   Merck, Darmstadt, Germany
pro analysis

Ampicillin trihydrate research grade	Serva Feinbiochemica, Heidelberg, Germany
Acetic acid 100 % (glacial) pro analysis	Merck, Darmstadt, Germany
_-D-Glucose	Serva Feinbiochemica, Heidelberg, Germany
AG® 501-x8 Resin	Bio-Rad Laboratories, Hercules, CA, USA
Boric Acid analytical grade	Serva Electrophoresis, Heidelberg, Germany
Calcium chloride	Merck, Darmstadt, Germany
Chloramphenicol chrystalline	Sigma-Aldrich, Vienna, Austria
Chloroform	Merck, Darmstadt,Germany
CTAB Hexadecyltrimethyl Ammonium Bromide	Sigma-Aldrich, Vienna, Austria
Dimethylsulfoxide (DMSO) for spectroscopy	Merck, Darmstadt, Germany
EDTA / Titriplex III	Merck, Darmstadt, Germany
Ethanol absolute pro analysis	Merck, Darmstadt, Germany
Ethidium Bromide Tablets 10 mg per tablet	Sigma Chemical Co, St. Louis, MO, USA

Ficoll 400	Sigma-Aldrich, Vienna, Austria
Dextran Sulfate 500 sodium salt stabilized	Serva Electrophoresis, Heidelberg, Germany
Formaldehyde solution 37 % for molecular biology	Merck, Darmstadt, Germany
Formamide pro analysis	Merck, Darmstadt, Germany
Glycerol 87 % pro analysis	Merck, Darmstadt, Germany
Hydrochloric acid, fuming 37 % pro analysis	Merck, Darmstadt, Germany
Isopropyl-1-thio-D-galactoside (IPTG)	Serva Electrophoresis, Heidelberg, Germany
Isoamyl alcohol GR pro analysis	Merck, Darmstadt, Germany
Isopropyl alcohol for chromotography	Merck, Darmstadt, Germany
Kanamycin monosulfate	Sigma-Aldrich, Vienna, Austria
LB-Broth, Miller	Difco Laboratories, Detroit, MI, USA
LB-Agar, Miller	Difco Laboratories, Detroit, MI, USA
Magnesium chloride	Merck, Darmstadt, Germany

2-Mercaptoethanol GR pro analysis	Merck, Darmstadt, Germany
Morpholinopropane sulfanic acid (MOPS)	Sigma-Aldrich, Vienna, Austria
Phenol:Chloroform:Isoamylalcohol (25:24:1 / V:V)	Gibco BRL, Life Technologies, Paisley, Scotland
Polyethylene Glycol 8000 (PEG)	Sigma-Aldrich, Vienna, Austria
Polyvinylpyrrolidone for molecular biology	Merck, Darmstadt, Germany
Potassium chloride pro analysis	Merck, Darmstadt, Germany
Potassium hydroxide Pellets pro analysis	Merck, Darmstadt, Germany
(di)-Potassium hydrogen phosphate pro analysis	Merck, Darmstadt, Germany
Potassium dihydrogen phosphate pro analysis	Merck, Darmstadt, Germany
Potassium hydrogen phosphate trihydrate pro analysis	Merck, Darmstadt, Germany
Qualex Gold Agarose	Hybaid AGS, Heidelberg, Germany
Rotiphenol (aqua-) for separation of RNA	Roth, Karlsruhe, Germany
RPMI 1640 Medium 1x	Seramed. Biomed, Berlin, Germany

Sodium-Dodecylsulfate, sodium salt 2x cryst. analytical grade	Serva Feinbiochemica, Heidelberg, Germany
Scintillation Cocktail Ready Safe™	Beckman Instruments, USA
Sodium acetate	Sigma-Aldrich, Vienna, Austria
Sodium bicarbonate	Merck, Darmstadt, Germany
Sodium chloride	Merck, Darmstadt, Germany
Sodium hydroxide pellets	Sigma-Aldrich, Vienna, Austria
Sodium pyrophosphate dehydrate	Merck, Darmstadt, Germany
Sucrose for molecular biology	Merck, Darmstadt, Germany
Tetracycline Hydrochloride	Serva Electrophoresis, Heidelberg, Germany
Tryptone Peptone pancreatic digest of casein	Difco Laboratories, Detroit, MI, USA
Tris (hydroxymethyl) aminomethane	Merck, Darmstadt, Germany
Tri-sodium-citrate dihydrate	Serva Electrophoresis, Heidelberg, Germany
Triton X-100	Serva Electrophoresis, Heidelberg, Germany

X-Gal/5-bromo-4-chloro-3-indolyl-beta-   Serva Electrophoresis, Heidelberg, Germany
D-galactoside, research grade

X-VIVO 20   Bio Whittaker, Walkerville, MD, USA

Xylene cyanol FF   Serva Electrophoresis, Heidelberg, Germany

Yeast extract   OXOID LTD, Basing stoke, Hampshire,
                                             Endland

4. Molecular Biology Tools

Advantage®-GC Genomic Polymerase   Clontech, Palo Alto, CA, USA
Mix

Alkaline Phosphatase   Serva Electrophoresis, Heidelberg, Germany
from calf intestine

Ampl Taq Gold^{TM} 5 U/µl   Perkin Elmar, Vienna, Austria
supplied, with 10x PCR buffer + MgCl$_2$

(_-^{32}P) dCTP   NEN, Boston, USA
3.000 Ci/mmol, 10 m Ci/ml

0.1 M DTT   Gibco BRL, Life Technologies, Paisley,
                                             Scotland

100 mM dATP   Promega, Madison, WI, USA

100 mM dCTP   Promega, Madison, WI, USA

100 mM dGTP	Promega, Madison, WI, USA
100 mM dTTP	Promega, Madison, WI, USA
Exonuclease III, 200 U/µl supplied ExoIII 10x buffer	Promega, Madison, WI, USA
Delta Tth DNA Polymerase Sequencing Kit	Clontech, Palo Alto, CA, USA
Deoxyribonucleic acid (from salmon testes)	Sigma Chemicals CO, St. Louis, MO, USA
Gene Ruler™, 100 bp DNA Ladder plus 0.5 mg DNA/ ml	MBI Fermentas, Vilnius, Lithuania
Gene Ruler™, 1 kb DNA Ladder 0.5 mg DNA/ml	MBI Fermentas, Vilnius, Lithuania
Lysozyme from chicken egg	Serva Electrophoresis, Heidelberg, Germany
Nucleobond 100 Kit	Macherey Nagel GmbH, Düren, Germany
Mouse Genome Walking Kit	Clontech, Palo Alto, CA, USA
Oligo-(dT)$_{15}$-Primer 0.5 mg/µl	Promega, Madison, WI, USA
pBluescript® II SK$^-$ Vector	Stratagene, La Jolla, CA, USA
pGL3 Basic-Vector	Promega, Madison, WI, USA

pGL3 Promoter-Vector   Promega, Madison, WI, USA

pRL-TK-Vector   Promega, Madison, WI, USA

Primers   Microsynth, Balgach, Switzerland

DNA Polymerase I Klenow-Fragment Promega, Madison, WI, USA
5 U/µl

Pfu-DNA Polymerase 3 U/µl   Promega, Madison, WI, USA
supplied Pfu 10x Rxn buffer

Proteinase K, solution (15.6 mg/ml) Boehringer Mannheim, Germany
in 10 mM Tris-HCl; pH 7.5

Quick Change™ Site-Directed   Stratagene, La Jolla, CA, USA
Mutagenesis Kit

QIAquick Gel Extraction Kit   Qiagen Inc., Valencia, CA, USA

QIAquick Nucleotide Removal Kit Qiagen Inc., Valencia, CA, USA

Random Hexamers   Promega, Madison, WI, USA
500 µl/ml

Restriction enzymes   Promega, Madison, WI, USA
supplied: 10x working buffers

RNasin®, 40 U/µl   Serva Electrophoresis, Heidelberg, Germany
Recombinant Ribonuclease Inhibitor

S1 Nuclease, 3 U/µl   Promega, Madison, WI, USA
supplied, with S1 Nuclease 10x
reaction buffer

Superscript II RT, 200 U/µl supplied, with 5x first strand buffer	Gibco BRL. Life Technologies, Paisley, Scotland
T4 DNA-Ligase 3 U/µl supplied, with T4 DNA-Ligase buffer 10x	Promega, Madison, WI, USA
Taq-Polymerase, 5 U/µl supplied, with Mg-free 10x buffer + $MgCl_2$ 25 mM	Promega, Madison, WI, USA
TaqStart[TM] Andibody 1.1 µg/µl	Clontech, Palo Alto, CA, USA
TOPO TA Cloning®-Kit	Invitrogen Corporation, Carlsbad, CA, USA

5. Materials

Bottle Top Filter 500 ml 0.22 µm Cellulose Acetate Sterilizing	Corning Costar, NY, USA
Duralon-UV[TM] Membranes 300x 30 cm/roll	Stratagene, La Jolla, CA, USA
Centrifuge Tube with Double Seal Cap, 15 ml, sterile	Iwaki Glass, Japan
Centrifuge Tube, 50 ml, sterile Polypropylene, disposable	Corning, NY, USA
Folded filters 595$^1/_2$, Ø 185 mm	Schleicher & Schuell, Dassel, Germany

Gloves latex for examinations	Sempermed, Semperit, Austria
Inoculating Needles disposable, sterile	Nunc, Brand Products, Germany
Kodak X-OMAT LS 32x 43 cm	Eastman Kodak Company, Rochester, NY, USA
Microcentrifuge tubes, 1.5 ml	Brand, Germany
Microcentrifuge tubes, 2 ml	Brand, Germany
Microtube, 1.5 ml, sterile	Sarstedt, Nümbrecht, Germany
Millipore, Filtertype:VS Pore size: 0.025 µM	Millipore Corporation, Bedford, MA, USA
Minisart; single-use filter unit, (0.20 µm) sterile, non-pyrogenic	Satorius AG, Göttingen, Germany
Petri Dish, sterile, Falcon Ten-twenty-nine ™	Becton Dickinson, Labware, NJ, USA
Polaroid Type 667, Coaterless Black and White Instant Pack Film	Polaroid Corporation, Cambridge, MA, USA
Pipettes, sterile disposable plastic a 5 ml, 10 ml, 25 ml, 50 ml	Bibby Sterilin, Stone, Staffordshire, England
Pipette tips, non-sterile, Plasticbrand® a 10 µl, 100 µl, 1000 µl	Brand, Germany
Pipette tips plus filter, 0.1-10 µl, sterile, non-pyrogenic, RNase/DNase free	Scientific Specialities, INC Lodi, CA, USA

Pipette tips plus filter, 1-200 µl, sterile, non-pyrogenic, RNase/DNase free	Corning, NY, USA
Pipette tips plus filter, 1000 µl, sterile	ART
Pasteur Pipettes, 230 mm length	Fortuna
Razor blades	Wilkinson Sword, Solingen, Germany
Round-Bottom Tube, 14 ml, sterile, non-pyrogenic	Falcon, Becton-Dickinson, NJ, USA
Saran, food wrap	Dow Chemical Company
Syringe 50 ml, sterile, non-pyrogenic; Plastipack	Becton-Dickinson, NJ, USA
Vial; Poly-Q; 18 ml	Beckman Instruments, USA
Thermowell^{TM} Tubes, 0.2 ml with Dome Cap, RNase/DNase free	Corning, NY, USA
96 Well Flat Bottom UV Plate, non-sterile	Costar, NY, USA
Whatman, Chromatography paper, 3 mm Chr	Whatman, Maidstone, England

6. Equipment

Blotter: Vacu-Blot System	Biometra, Göttingen, Germany
Camera: Polaroid DS 34 direct screen instant camera	Polaroid Corporation, Cambridge, MA, USA
Centrifuge: Omnifuge 2.0 RS	Heraeus Intruments, Hanau, Germany
Centrifuge: Cryofuge 5000	Heraeus Intruments, Hanau, Germany
Centrifuge: Sorvall® RC Plus	Du Pont, Vienna, Austria
Centrifuge: MP4R Centra®	IEC International Equipment Company
Centrifuge: Biofuge fresco	Heraeus Intruments, Hanau, Germany
Centrifuge: Microfuge^{TM} 12	Beckman Instruments, Fullerton, CA, USA
Distiller: Destamat Bi 18 E	Heraeus Quarzglas, Hanau, Germany
Exposure Cassette (Phosphoimager)	Molecular Dynamics
Gelelectrophoresis Mini Submarine Agarose Gel Unit HE33	Hoefer Scientific Instruments, San Francisco, CA, USA
Gelelectorphoresis MAX Submarine Agarose Gel Unit / Model HE99	Hoefer Scientific Instruments, San Francisco, CA, USA

Hybridisation Oven (mini)	Biometra, Göttingen, Germany
Hybridisation tubes HB-OV-BL	Hybaid, Middlesex, England
Incubator BM400	Memmbert GmbH, Schwabach Germany
Microwave, Rowenta MW 22	Rowenta, Germany
PCR: GeneAmp PCR System 2 400	Perkin Elmer, Vienna, Austria
PCR: GeneAmp PCR System 9 600	Perkin Elmer, Vienna, Austria
pH-Meter E512	Metrohm Herisau, Switzerland
Power Supply GPS 200/400, PP 3000 Programmable High Voltage Power Pack	Biometra, Göttingen, Germany
Pipettes 0.5-10 µl Eppendorf Reference® variable	Eppendorf-Netheler-Hinz-GmbH, Hamburg; Germany
Pipettes 10-100 µl Eppendorf Reference® variable	Eppendorf-Netheler-Hinz-GmbH, Hamburg, Germany
Pipettes 100-1000 µl Eppendorf Reference® variable	Eppendorf-Netheler-Hinz-GmbH, Hamburg; Germany
Pipetboy Accu-Pipette	IBC Integra Biosciences
Scale: Weight Basic plus (BP)	Sartorius, Rattingen, Germany

Scanner: Storm 840	Molecular Dynamics
Scintillation Counter (multi-purpose) LS 6500	Beckman Instruments, USA
Shaker: GFL 3032	GFL-Gesellschaft für Labortechnik, Burgwedel, Germany
Spectrophometer for microplate scanning Lambda Scan 200	Bio-Tek Instruments, Winoosik, VT, USA
Storage Phosphor Screen 20 x 25 cm	Molecular Dynamics
Storm 840 scanner	Molecular Dynamics
Stratalinker Stratagene® UV Stratalinker 2400	Stratagene, Vienna, Austria
Tube Heater SHT 1	Stuart Scientific, U.K.
UV-Transilluminator, 2011 Macrovue LBB	UVP.INC, San Gabriel, CF, USA
Vortex: VF2	Janke+Kunkle IKA® Labortechnik Staufen, Germany
Water Bath: Julabo TWB6 / 5 / SW-20C	Julabo Labortechnik GmbH, Salbach, Germany

Curriculum vitae

Mag. rer. nat. Martina Meyer

Personal Data

Date of Birth	July 10, 1972
Place of Birth	Innsbruck/Austria
Citizenship	Austria

Scientific Education

1987-91	Secondary School in Innsbruck /Austria
1991-94	**Undergraduate study in Biology**; (1st Diploma) Leopold Franzens University of Innsbruck/Austria
1994-98	**Undergraduate study in Microbiology**; (2nd Diploma) extended in the fields of Molecular Biology, Medical Biochemistry and Immunology
1996-98	***M.S. Thesis*** "Characterization of 6-pyruvoyl-tetrahydropterin-synthase messenger RNA from human myelomonocytoma cell line THP-1" Institute of Medical Chemistry and Biochemistry, University of Innsbruck, Austria; Supervisor: A.Prof. Dr. Ernst Werner
since 1998	***Ph.D. Thesis*** "Genomic characterization of the T-cell activating CXC-chemokine SCYB11 from man and mouse" Institute of Medical Chemistry and Biochemistry, University of Innsbruck, Austria; Supervisor: A.Prof. Dr. Gabriele Werner-Felmayer

Publications

Original papers

Laich A, **Meyer M**, Werner ER, Werner-Felmayer G: Structure and expression of the human small cytokine B subfamily member 11 (SCYB11/formerly SCYB9B, alias I-TAC) gene cloned from IFN-_-treated human monocytes (THP-1). J Interferon Cytokine Res. 19: 505-513 (1999)

Meyer M, Erdel M, Duba HC, Werner ER, Werner-Felmayer G: Cloning, genomic sequence, and chromosome mapping of SCYB11, the murine homologue of *Scyb11* (alias _R1/H174/SCYB9B9/I-TAC/CXCL11). Cytogenet Cell Genet. 88: 278-282 (2000)

Meyer M, Tensen CP, Hensbergen PJ, van der Raaij-Helmer E, Brandacher G, Margreiter R, Heufler C, Koch F, Narumi S, Werner ER, Colvin R, Luster AD, Tensen CP, Werner-Felmayer G: Cross reactivity of three T-cell attracting murine chemokines stimulating the CXC chemokine receptor CXCR3 and their induction in cultured cells and during allograpft rejection, submitted

Erdel M, Theurl M, **Meyer M**, Duba HD, Utermann G, Werner-Felmayer G: High-Resolution Mapping of the Human 4q21 and the Murine 5E3 SCYB Chemokine Cluster by Fiber-FISH, submitted

in preparation

Leitner K, **Meyer M**, Werner ER, Leimbacher W, Thöny B, Werner-Felmayer G: Tetrahydrobiopterin Biosynthesis in human monocytes: Splicing variants of 6-pyruvoyl tetrahydropterin synthase mRNA

Meyer M, Werner ER, Werner-Felmayer G: Human and murine SCYB11: Analysis of the promoter activity

Book contributions

Meyer M, Werner-Felmayer G, Werner ER, Heufler-Tiefenthaler C, Thöny B, Leimbacher W: Characterization of 6-pyruvoly tetrahydropterin synthase messenger RNA from myelomonocytic THP-1 cells. In: Chemistry and Biology of Pteridines and Folates 1997 (Eds. Pfleiderer W, Rokos H) Blackwell Science Berlin, Vienna, Oxford, Edinburgh, Boston, London, Melbourne, Paris, Tokyo; pp 623-625 (1997)

Werner-Felmayer G, **Meyer M**, Werner ER: Cytokine-induced pteridine biosynthesis in human monocytes (THP-1): Analysis of its molecular basis. In: Chemistry and Biology of Pteridines and Folates 1997 (Eds. Pfleiderer W, Rokos H) Blackwell Science Berlin, Vienna, Oxford, Edinburgh, Boston, London, Melbourne, Paris, Tokyo; pp 585-590 (1997)

Abstracts

Meyer M, Werner-Felmayer G, Heufler-Tiefenthaler C, Leimbacher W, Wachter H, Thöny B, Werner ER: Characterization of 6-pyruvoyl tetrahydropterin synthase messenger RNA from human myelomonocytic THP-1 cells. Pteridines 7: 73 (1997)

Meyer M, Werner-Felmayer G, Heufler-Tiefenthaler C, Leimbacher W, Wachter H, Thöny B, Werner E: Characterization of 6-pyruvoyl tetrahydropterin synthase messenger RNA from human myelomonocytic THP-1 cells. Pteridines 8: 41 (1997)

Werner-Felmayer G, Plüss C, Leimbacher W, **Meyer M**, Heufler-Tiefenthaler C, Pfeilschifter J, Thöny B, Wachter H, Werner ER: Cytokine-induced pteridines biosynthesis in human monocytes (THP-1): Analysis of its molecular basis. Pteridines 8: 60 (1997)

Meyer M, Werner-Felmayer G, Heufler-Tiefenthaler C, Thöny B, Leimbacher W, Werner ER: Relative abundance of 6-pyruvoyl tetrahydrobiopterin synthase mRNA species in human monocytes, macrophages and fibroblasts. Pteridines 9: 156 (1998)

Meyer M, Erdel M, Duba H, Theurl M, Werner ER, Werner-Felmayer G: Molecular comparison of human and murine SCYB11. Europ. Cytokine Network 11: 121 (2000)

Werner-Felmayer G, van der Raaij-Helmer EMH, Hensbergen PH, **Meyer M**, Werner ER, Tensen CP: Expression patterns and bioactivity of murine SCYB11 (muSCYB11). Europ. Cytokine Network 11: 119 (2000)

Poster presentations

Meyer M, Werner-Felmayer G, Werner ER, Heufler-Tiefenthaler C, Thöny B, Leimbacher W. Institute for Medical Chemistry and Biochemistry, University of Innsbruck, Austria; Characterization of 6-pyruvolytetrahydropterin synthase messenger RNA from myelomonocytic THP-1 cells; *11th International Symposium on Chemistry and Biology of Pteridines and Folates, Berchtesgaden*, **Germany (1997)**

Meyer M, Laich A, Werner ER, Werner-Felmayer G. Institute for Medical Chemistry and Biochemistry, University of Innsbruck, Austria. Molecular characterization of human small cytokine B subfamily member 9beta (SCYB9B) *Keystone Symposia on Molecular & Cellular Biology / Chemokines and Chemokine Receptors, Keystone,Colorado,* **USA (1999)**

Meyer M, Erdel M, Theurl M, Werner ER, Werner-Felmayer G. Institute for Medical Chemistry and Biochemistry and Institute of Medical Biology University of Innsbruck, Innsbruck, Austria; Comparison of the T-cell activation CXC chemokine SCYB11 from man and mouse; *Annual conference of Austrian Biochemical Society and Austrian Society for Genetic.* **Innsbruck, Austria (2000)**

Meyer M, Erdel M, Duba H, Theurl M, Werner ER, Werner-Felmayer G. Institute for Medical Chemistry and Biochemistry and Institute of Medical Biology University of Innsbruck, Innsbruck, Austria; Molecular comparison of human and murine SCYB11; *3rd Join Meeting of the International Cytokine Society (ICS) and the International Society for Interferon and Cytokine Research (ISICR).* **Amsterdam, Netherlands (2000)**

Acknowledgements

First of all I want to thank my supervisor <u>Dr. Gabriele Werner-Felmayer</u> for giving me the opportunity to work on this project and for guiding me through in a very supportive and friendly manner.

Special thanks also to <u>Dr. Ernst Werner</u> for his scientific advice and his countless supports.

Moreover, words of thanks to <u>all people in our lab</u> for their countless helps and essential contributions to this work.

Particularly I want to mention <u>Petra Höfler</u>, who generously helped me by doing all cell culture work, <u>Mag. Anja Peterbauer</u>, who carried out the LAL-test and assisted me with the data interpretation in Excel, and <u>Renate Kaus,</u> who inaugurated me in all Molecular Biological skills. To all three also special thanks for patiently answering my numerous questions.

Furthermore, a warm thank you to <u>Dr. Martin Spitaler</u> for his assistance with transfection and to <u>Dr. Martin Erdel</u> for his valuable contributions concerning the gene organization.

I am also grateful to <u>my parents</u> who enabled me the study and encouraged me in various ways and also to <u>Thomas Kurz</u> for this mental support.